Performance Improvement: Winning Strategies for Quality and JCAHO Compliance
Second Edition

Cynthia Barnard, MM, CPHQ
Jodi L. Eisenberg, CMSC

OPUS COMMUNICATIONS
A Division of *hc*Pro

Performance Improvement: Winning Strategies for Quality and JCAHO Compliance, Second Edition, is published by Opus Communications, a division of HCPro.

Copyright 2000 Opus Communications, a division of HCPro.

All rights reserved. Printed in the United States of America.   5   4   3   2   1

ISBN 1-57839-089-3

No part of this publication may be reproduced, in any form or by any means, without prior written consent of Opus Communications or the Copyright Clearance Center (978/750-8400). Please notify us immediately if you have received an unauthorized copy.

Opus Communications provides information resources for the health care industry.

A selected listing of our newsletters and books is found at the back of this book.

Opus Communications is not affiliated in any way with the Joint Commission on Accreditation of Healthcare Organizations.

Cynthia Barnard, MM, CPHQ, & Jodi Eisenberg, CMSC, Authors
John Hoffacker, Editor
Jean St. Pierre, Creative Director
Thomas Philbrook, Cover Designer
Rob Stuart, Publisher
Jennifer Cofer, RRA, Executive Publisher
Silverchair Science + Communications, Inc., production

Advice given is general. Readers should consult professional counsel for specific legal, ethical, or clinical questions.

Arrangements can be made for quantity discounts. For more information contact:
Opus Communications
P.O. Box 1168
Marblehead, MA 01945
Telephone: 800/650-6787 or 781/639-1872
Fax: 781/639-2982
E-mail: customer_service@hcpro.com
www.hcpro.com, www.hcmarketplace.com, www.accreditinfo.com

Dedicated to
Rebecca, Sarah Bethany,
Daniel, and Kaitlyn

Contents

Figures ix
About the Authors xi
Acknowledgments xiii
Preface xv
Introduction xvii

Part I   Meeting Basic JCAHO Requirements

Chapter 1   Making Sense of the JCAHO's Performance Improvement Standards 3

    PI.1: Developing your performance improvement plan 4
    PI.2: Designing your performance improvement approach 7
    PI.3: Collecting and measuring data 10
    PI.4: Evaluating data 16
    PI.5: Making improvements 19

Chapter 2   Understanding Other Standards Related to Performance Improvement 21

    JCAHO's patient-focused standards 21
    Leadership (LD) 24
    Environment of care (EC) 26
    Human resources (HR) 28
    Information management (IM) 29
    Surveillance, prevention, and control of infection (IC) 31
    Medical staff (MS) 32
    Governance (GO), management (MA), and nursing (NR) 34

Chapter 3   The ORYX Initiative and Core Performance Measures: New Challenges for Your Hospital 37

    What is ORYX? 37
    Participating in ORYX 37
    Challenges of ORYX and the core measures 38
    Selecting a performance measurement system 38
    Introducing the core performance measurement initiative 43

Part II Managing the Performance Improvement Process

Chapter 4 *Preparing for Survey: The Key Is an Organized, Ongoing, and Consistent Approach* 47

    Opening conference and performance improvement overview session 48
    Document review session 52
    Leadership interviews 53
    Performance improvement team interview 58
    Performance improvement coordinating group interview 60
    Interviews with hospital staff 61
    Environment of care document review and interview sessions 64
    Resource management interview 66
    Conclusion 68

Chapter 5 *Leadership's Role in Performance Improvement* 69

    Leadership performance improvement cycle 70
    Individual leaders' performance improvement responsibilities 71

Chapter 6 *Implementing the Performance Improvement Plan: The Performance Improvement Director's Role* 83

    Where to focus and how fast to move 83
    Creating a sound performance improvement infrastructure 87
    Conducting departmental self-evaluations 88
    Forms and information flow 88
    Implementing the program 89
    Overseeing your performance improvement program's data collection 95
    Designing data collection 96
    Establishing performance improvement training programs 99
    Monitoring implementation of performance improvement throughout the hospital 100
    Other responsibilities of performance improvement directors 101

Chapter 7 *Working Successfully with Performance Improvement Teams* 105

    When do you need a performance improvement team? 106
    Selecting a performance improvement team model 106
    Choosing performance improvement team members and chartering the team .. 108
    Training task teams on the performance improvement model 110
    Supporting your performance improvement teams 112
    Guiding performance improvement teams through the "Plan, Design, Measure, Assess, and Improve" process 115
    Analyzing the performance improvement team's results 118
    Dealing with a team's failure 118

Part III Understanding the Performance Improvement Process

Chapter 8 *The Blueprint for Success: Developing Your Hospital's Performance Improvement Plan (PI.1)* 121

    Defining your performance improvement approach 122

Setting improvement priorities 125
Defining the audience for your performance improvement plan 126
Developing the performance improvement plan 126
Distributing the performance improvement plan 131

Chapter 9 Designing New Processes and Programs (PI.2) 133

Why is it important to design new processes in accordance with
performance improvement principles? 133
Incorporating JCAHO design requirements into your business planning
and performance improvement frameworks 134
Documenting the design of a process 134

**Chapter 10 Performance Measurement: The Key to Your Performance Improvement
Program's Success (PI.3)** 135

Why measure at all? 135
Meeting JCAHO standards 136
Measuring other JCAHO-required elements 137
Benchmarking and ORYX/core measure requirements: other considerations
in designing and selecting measures 148
Linking your measures to the hospital's strategic goals 149
Managing the measurement process 149

Chapter 11 Assessing Your Results: Where Do You Go from Here? (PI. 4) 153

Who conducts assessments? 154
Comparing gathered data with JCAHO-required comparative data 154
Identifying sentinel events and "bad apples" 155
Documenting assessments 157
Reporting your results to the quality oversight committee 158
Conducting the hospital-wide performance improvement assessment 159

Chapter 12 The Final Stage: Implementing Improvements (PI. 5) 161

Establishing your improvement priorities 162
Designing your improvement plan 164
Implementing improvements 164
Documenting your actions 165
Conducting the annual hospital-wide appraisal 171
External rewards for an outstanding performance improvement program ... 176

Appendix 1 Pre-Survey Checklist: Accreditation Requirements for Performance Improvement 179

Appendix 2 Pre-Survey Checklist: ORYX Compliance 183

Appendix 3 Pre-Survey Checklist: Sentinel Events 184

Bibliography 187

Annotated List of Healthcare Quality-Related Web Sites 189

Figures

Figure 1.1	Demonstrating integration among strategic, operational, and quality planning	6
Figure 1.2	Summary of required measures	11
Figure 1.3	Considering measures for discontinuation	12
Figure 3.1	Making the first cut: which vendors' systems should you evaluate?	39
Figure 3.2	Evaluating your "short list": choosing the one performance measurement system that's right for you	40
Figure 4.1	Preparing for the performance improvement overview presentation	49
Figure 4.2	Performance improvement documentation	54
Figure 4.3	Sample questions and answers for leaders	56
Figure 4.4	The mock survey	62
Figure 4.5	Mock survey assessment checklist	63
Figure 4.6	Mock survey interviews	65
Figure 5.1	Governing board performance improvement compliance checklist	73
Figure 5.2	Establishing a quality oversight committee	74
Figure 5.3	Model agenda for quality oversight committee	75
Figure 5.4	Senior managers' performance improvement compliance checklist	76
Figure 5.5	Performance improvement director's performance improvement compliance checklist	77
Figure 5.6	Medical staff leaders' performance improvement compliance checklist	79
Figure 5.7	Line operations managers' performance improvement compliance checklist	80
Figure 6.1	Monitoring current trends	85
Figure 6.2	Conducting a departmental performance improvement self-assessment	89
Figure 6.3	Identifying a department's performance improvement priorities	90
Figure 6.4	Planning for measurement	91
Figure 6.5	Measurement data report	92

Figures

Figure 6.6	Orientation to performance improvement planning for managers and medical leaders	93
Figure 6.7	Outline of a performance improvement training handbook for managers	94
Figure 6.8	What the hospital's performance improvement director should know about data collection and evaluation	96
Figure 6.9	Agenda for performance improvement orientation of new employees	101
Figure 6.10	The "red card game" leader guide	102
Figure 7.1	Sample performance improvement team charter	109
Figure 7.2	Outline of a "just in time" performance improvement training workshop	111
Figure 7.3	Sample "just in time" performance improvement training workshop agenda	112
Figure 7.4	Outline of a "How to lead a performance improvement team" workshop	113
Figure 7.5	Common performance improvement tools	114
Figure 7.6	Performance improvement team action plans	116
Figure 8.1	Matching your performance improvement model to the JCAHO's Plan, Design, Measure, Assess, Improve model	123
Figure 8.2	Selecting a performance improvement model	124
Figure 8.3	Northwestern Memorial Hospital's performance improvement plan outline	128
Figure 10.1	How a performance improvement project meets JCAHO requirements	138
Figure 10.2	Mapping performance improvement measurements to JCAHO requirements	139
Figure 10.3	Core elements of the JCAHO's sentinel event policy	148
Figure 10.4	Samples of compliance with JCAHO measurement requirements	151
Figure 11.1	Reporting hierarchy	159
Figure 12.1	Performance improvement team progress report	167
Figure 12.2	Performance improvement team workbook contents	168
Figure 12.3	Sample presentation	169
Figure 12.4	Performance improvement team and departmental self-assessment	172
Figure 12.5	Request for information on annual performance improvement achievements	174
Figure 12.6	Annual performance improvement program assessment	175
Figure 12.7	Outline of a performance improvement program annual assessment	176

About the Authors

Cynthia Barnard, MM, CPHQ, is the director for quality strategies and safety at Northwestern Memorial Hospital, an affiliate of Northwestern University Medical School. She is responsible for quality improvement, patient satisfaction measurement and improvement, accreditation and regulatory compliance, and safety. In recent years, she took a leadership role in developing the healthcare standards for the Lincoln Foundation for Business Excellence, an Illinois equivalent to the national Malcolm Baldrige business excellence award.

Prior roles at Northwestern and elsewhere have included direction of medical staff affairs and clinical research, and developing and consulting on healthcare information systems for operational support and strategic planning and analysis. She holds a master's degree in management from Northwestern University's Kellogg School of Management, a bachelor's degree in psychology from Bryn Mawr College, and the Certified Professional in Healthcare Quality designation from the National Association for Healthcare Quality.

Jodi L. Eisenberg, CMSC, is coordinator of accreditation and licensure at Northwestern Memorial Hospital in Chicago, Illinois, and an editorial advisor for Executive Briefings on Hospital Regulations, published by Opus Communications. She received a bachelor's degree in healthcare administration at the University of St. Francis. During her 14 years in healthcare, Jodi has worked primarily in the field of medical staff services, focusing on management and consulting with expertise in credentialing, medical staff privileging, quality management, medical staff organization, and JCAHO accreditation standards.

In her current role, she is responsible for leading the full range of JCAHO and other accreditation and regulatory compliance activities, including organization of preparation activities for JCAHO and other site surveys. Her hospital scored in the top 1% of hospitals nationally in a recent JCAHO survey.

Acknowledgments

We are indebted to a number of important people for their assistance in teaching us, giving us the opportunity to test our own theories about effective PI, and supporting us as we wrote this book.

First, we want to thank John Hoffacker, our editor, whose thoughtful comments helped us improve the manuscript.

We also thank the senior management team at Northwestern Memorial Hospital, where we are both employed, for their exceptional support in developing a successful and rewarding PI program—particularly Kathleen Murray, executive vice president; Lawrence Michaelis, MD, senior vice president for medical affairs; Loretta Alexander, administrative coordinator; and others at Northwestern Memorial who have been consistently helpful in developing the program.

And, as a couple of working moms with busy lives, we thank our families for their patience while we devoted "their" time to writing, rewriting, and re-rewriting.

Preface

This book is designed to help you do more than just meet Joint Commission on Accreditation of Healthcare Organizations (JCAHO) performance improvement (PI) requirements; it offers you sound, easy-to-implement, practical advice on how to develop a PI program that effectively improves the quality of care in your hospital. Each chapter clearly describes what is required by the JCAHO, what is optional and/or likely to become a future requirement, and what important issues beyond the standards you should consider.

Chapters 1, 2, 3, and **4** provide an overview of all the standards directly or indirectly related to PI in the JCAHO's *Comprehensive Accreditation Manual for Hospitals (CAMH)*. They describe

- The JCAHO's formal requirements
- What surveyors really want to see
- What documents you should prepare
- How you can prepare for the PI interview
- Which questions surveyors might ask
- How you can ensure your PI program is compliant
- How to meet the JCAHO's new ORYX and core performance measurement requirements

Chapters 5, 6, and **7** offer advice on how to manage the PI process. These chapters describe the roles of key hospital leaders such as your governing body, senior leaders, medical staff leaders, and line managers in your PI program. They also will teach you the role of the PI director in the improvement process and how to manage PI teams effectively.

Chapter 8 outlines a methodical, comprehensive approach to the development and documentation of a PI plan for your hospital that meets JCAHO standards and will genuinely advance your PI program.

Chapter 9 briefly discusses some simple steps you can take to ensure that the design of your PI programs complies with JCAHO requirements.

Preface

Chapter 10 speaks to one of the most confusing and problematic topics in PI—the development of a complete list of measurements that meet the extensive requirements of the PI chapter in the *CAMH*. When you work through this chapter, you will have a straightforward approach to inventorying and evaluating your measurements to ensure that you are indeed in full compliance with these standards.

Chapter 11 helps you with the all-important task of assessing the data that your departments and teams have collected, ensuring that you meet the JCAHO's requirements for thorough analysis.

Chapter 12 concludes the PI cycle with a focus on improvement, including an overview of how to collect and document an annual summary of the outcomes of your PI program, which is also required for full compliance.

We have been actively involved in hospital PI and JCAHO compliance for more than 18 years between us, and we understand exactly how difficult it is to develop and maintain a PI program. The best single piece of advice we can offer you is to focus on what really matters to your hospital and then to use the JCAHO standards to help you stay rigorously organized and ensure that your program genuinely serves your patients and your community.

In other words, the JCAHO standards are a means to an end. Compliance should be so fully woven into every management and staff function that no staff members ever feel that they are working "to meet a JCAHO standard." Instead, they should feel that the standards offer a constructive framework to ensure that they are working "to improve patient care and support services."

As a leader, you can develop and sustain a program that accomplishes this. The initiatives of the JCAHO since the late 1980s, and particularly since the early 1990s, have produced a group of surveyors who are generally better trained, more sensitive to the needs and opportunities of today's hospitals, and better listeners than we have ever seen before. Our experience with these surveyors has been that a well-organized program with a clear structure, a meaningful link to hospital mission and vision, and demonstrable outcomes is a sure winner every time.

If "the devil is in the details," this book will help you take the bedevilment out of PI and ensure that the details are thoroughly addressed so that your program can keep its solid, vigorous focus on improving care and support for your patients and your community.

The book includes a large number of helpful figures and forms, many of which we have personally developed and reviewed with JCAHO surveyors. Although these are merely illustrations from selected settings, we believe that they will help make our recommendations clear and concrete and will give you a head start as you develop or enhance your own PI program.

We've enjoyed this project. We hope it delivers value to you, and we welcome your comments.

Cynthia Barnard, Director, Quality Strategies/Safety
Jodi Eisenberg, Coordinator, Accreditation and Licensure
Northwestern Memorial Hospital
Chicago, Illinois

Introduction

In today's healthcare environment, performance improvement (PI) is a business imperative, linked to effective competition and cost management. Healthcare organizations have discovered the same truth that returned other American industries to international competitiveness—high-quality processes are less expensive in the long run than poor-quality processes. They produce a more satisfied work force, fewer defects, less waste, and fewer lost customers. In healthcare, better processes produce better outcomes, and that means your patients and community benefit from better care, better health, and lower overall healthcare costs.

The objective of a PI program is to support a high level of patient care quality. A comprehensive program must protect patient and worker safety, effectively identify processes or individuals with quality problems, and continuously scan for opportunities to improve performance.

Many PI approaches have surfaced in healthcare recently, such as total quality management (TQM) or continuous quality improvement (CQI), only to fall from management favor due to excessively elaborate structures and unrealistic work force training goals. These initiatives focused heavily on process, with little attention to outcome. Too many TQM/CQI programs measured their success by how many people were trained, how many teams were formed, and how many hours were spent collecting and analyzing data, and not on performance itself. A flurry of articles in quality journals in the early 1990s had titles such as "Is Quality Dead?" and "The End of TQM." Businesses were beginning to recognize that they had allowed themselves to focus too much on the bureaucracy and process of quality and not enough on results and outcomes.

The Joint Commission's requirements

The Joint Commission on Accreditation of Healthcare Organizations (JCAHO) standards for PI offer hospitals what many past quality initiatives didn't: a focus on their core mission, the delivery of outstanding patient care. These standards, along with other quality recognition initiatives such as the federal Malcolm Baldrige quality assessment process and awards remind hospitals that, although it is important to have a comprehensive and thoughtful process, the sole purpose of PI is to improve actual performance! As you will see throughout this book, the JCAHO encourages hospitals to develop a PI program that focuses substantially on a few key issues rather than scattering energy among hundreds of minor efforts.

The standards also require leaders to make PI an integral part of the hospital's strategy and operations. These leadership and PI standards recognize and correct the single most common failing of most hospital PI programs—the idea that a PI program is separate from the rest of the hospital's goals and unconnected to key hospital operations, strategies, and relationships. Just a few years ago, the quality programs often measured quality indicators because they were convenient or of special interest. Today, leaders must ensure that staff measure indicators that are functionally related to clinical outcomes and drive patient or physician satisfaction. They must work to improve the performance of key processes in the hospital.

A significant insight drove the JCAHO to this new outlook on PI. It recognized that every quality measurement should be linked to the hospital's operational and strategic goals. Quality, then, is a product of well-designed and well-executed systems that respond to customer needs and use the talents of the entire work force. Performance is improved when systems are improved. Although some quality and performance problems are related to poor individual performance, this is a small percentage (perhaps 15%) that can be reduced by reevaluating the hiring, selection, and training systems.

Hospitals also need to monitor and improve performance through teamwork. Effective planning, design, and improvement can occur only when physicians, nurses, professionals, and support staff all work together toward a common goal. This insight is not new to hospitals, but it reflects the growing awareness of the need for collaborative relationships to produce high-quality patient care. It is also the recipe for reducing costs and improving patient care.

The benefits of PI

Why should a hospital devote energy to developing an outstanding PI program? Although the JCAHO does require you to have a competent PI system, this is not enough. We should develop an outstanding PI program because PI is at the core of the mission of every healthcare provider. Unless every hospital, nurse, physician, and healthcare professional is dedicated to improving the health of each patient and the community, we do not have a reason to exist.

Well-designed and well-implemented PI initiatives can result in improved patient health, reduced costs, a happier and more collaborative work force, heightened competitiveness, and a hospital that is generally better able to serve its community (even at a time when resources are severely restricted). Definitive research on the relationship of quality and PI to strategic success has yet to be performed, but the literature is replete with success stories of hospitals that have achieved market and strategic success in part through improved quality and value.

The JCAHO's new PI philosophy is both elegant and concise, particularly compared to more bureaucratic and process-focused forms of total quality management or continuous quality improvement. It maps easily to quality frameworks used in the larger business environment, such as Deming and Juran's strategies. And it is flexible enough to readily adapt to your hospital's needs and hold us all to high standards for quality.

Tougher JCAHO demands today and in the future

As we enter the twenty-first century, the healthcare quality profession is experiencing its most dramatic challenge since the redefinition of quality assurance into quality and PI 10 years ago. With the release of numerous studies linking performance variation and human-factors research with medical error and patient mortality and morbidity, we are challenged to use the accumulated knowledge and tools of PI to effect improvement in healthcare outcomes on an unprecedented scale.

The Institute of Medicine study on medical errors, released late in 1999, estimated that as many as 98,000 deaths per year were attributable to medical error (see Bibliography). Both that study and all the many responses and commentaries on it have emphasized the importance of systematic improvement of processes in reducing error.

The Joint Commission is well aware of these trends. In mid-1999 it sent a 10-minute videotape to the CEO of every accredited hospital that should be required viewing at senior quality committees. The videotape outlines changes that have already been enacted—such as expanded scope of random unannounced visits—and changes that will continue to evolve, such as an intensified focus on actual clinical outcomes, errors encountered and avoided, and systems thinking. The overriding message of the videotape, and of all JCAHO communications addressing PI and the accreditation process, has been accountability in a new and more challenging evolution.

In the 1999 and 2000 updates of its accreditation manual, the JCAHO intensified its demands on hospitals' PI programs not by adding or changing the standards but by lifting many scoring caps. Within the PI chapter, there are no scoring caps. In other words, failure now to comply with any standard in the PI section can result in a Type I recommendation.

To the problems of medical error and diffuse accountability for healthcare performance, well-designed and executed PI is not only one possible solution—national leaders in quality generally agree that it is the **only** solution (see Bibliography). The importance of the PI program guided by vigorous, thoughtful, and effective leadership has never been greater.

In short, the Joint Commission is holding us to a higher standard for PI than ever before. Surveyors will focus on improvement that is carefully planned, executed, and sustained. In addition, changes to the standard survey agenda will provide the surveyors with increased time during their visit to focus on hospital-specific issues. This increased time will almost certainly lead to the likelihood of increased recommendations requiring corrective action within the hospital and either a written progress report and/or a revisit. It is clearly in the hospital's best interest to avoid these recommendations by ensuring compliance with the standards before a survey occurs.

Furthermore, in light of the increased focus on medical error and error reduction in healthcare, most hospital governing boards want to see the increased accountability and clear definition of measurement of performance that are integral to a well-designed PI program. As a PI leader, you are in a position to respond to this new and dramatic dual challenge from both the national inquiry into error and the accreditation focus.

Part I

Meeting Basic JCAHO Requirements

Chapter 1

Making Sense of the JCAHO's Performance Improvement Standards

The Joint Commission on the Accreditation of Healthcare Organizations' (JCAHO) performance improvement (PI) standards are some of the most important standards in the *Comprehensive Accreditation Manual for Hospitals (CAMH)*—they are the cornerstone of the accreditation manual and the JCAHO's latest approach to accreditation. To provide patients with the best possible care, you need to consistently monitor, analyze, and, if necessary, improve all of the processes in your hospital that directly and indirectly affect patient care. The JCAHO's PI standards offer the guidelines you need to help you meet that goal.

Although all of the JCAHO's requirements, such as those for leadership, environment of care, and patient and family education, pose some challenges for hospitals, the PI standards have become a primary focus in healthcare nationwide. These standards present a challenge to your facility like none other. You need to demonstrate to your surveyors that PI truly is an organization-wide priority.

Although the JCAHO has issued relatively few type 1 recommendations for noncompliance with the PI standards for hospitals, the PI chapter remains as one of the most important in the *CAMH*, because it is so strongly linked to every other chapter in the book. Your best strategy is to have in place—long before surveyors arrive—an organized, ongoing, and consistent approach to PI.

You can expect your surveyors to review and assess your hospital's level of compliance with the PI standards in virtually every survey session on their agenda. To ensure that you meet their expectations, you need a clear understanding of what the standards mean and what the JCAHO wants from you. For example, standards PI.1 through PI.5 require you to

- Develop a hospital-wide PI plan.
- Establish a consistent and collaborative approach to PI.
- Collect and evaluate data according to specific JCAHO guidelines.
- Systematically document improvements achieved in your organization.

These requirements seem simple enough on the surface, but once you begin to develop and implement your hospital's PI plan and try to wade through the JCAHO's convoluted language and jargon, you'll probably develop a long list of questions that need answers.

Chapter 1

Read through this chapter to help you understand exactly what the JCAHO's requirements are and how you should apply them to your hospital. Each standard is dissected and explained in clear, understandable terms. Lists of key JCAHO-required documents and potential questions surveyors may ask will help you prepare your paperwork and staff for the surveyors' visit, and practical compliance tips will help you gauge whether your PI program is on track.

PI.1: Developing your performance improvement plan

JCAHO's requirements

Standards PI.1–PI.1.1 require your hospital leaders to develop a PI plan that describes exactly how the organization will identify opportunities for improvement in clinical and nonclinical systems. The plan should describe the collaborative strategy you've developed to assess and improve processes within the hospital, especially those that cross department lines. Your attention to interdisciplinary processes, such as medication orders, dispensing, and administration, demonstrates that your hospital takes a single approach to PI and applies it consistently across the organization.

An ideal comprehensive PI plan

1. Is consistent with the mission and vision of the hospital and individual departments
2. Includes a mechanism to receive input from internal and external customers
3. Requires the use of performance measurement tools
4. Encourages collaboration among all departments and disciplines in the hospital
5. Assures disciplined assessment, development of solutions, and maintenance of improvements
6. Provides flexibility to meet changing priorities
7. Suggests how to determine improvement priorities
8. Describes the improvement process in consistent use throughout the organization

What surveyors want

The surveyors will look for evidence that your managers constantly seek opportunities to improve all day-to-day operational issues, and they will expect them to offer examples of real improvements that have been made. For example, you might focus on improving chemotherapy administration or developing diagnosis-specific education plans. Although your PI plan is important to surveyors and necessary for you to achieve accreditation, proof that the organization has fully embraced your PI philosophy is just as critical.

Although surveyors will be most interested in multidisciplinary and hospital-wide improvement efforts, they still will want to see examples of department-specific improvement activities, such as improving radiology report turnaround times. These departmental improvement efforts should be consistent with the hospital's PI plan and should be interdisciplinary where and when appropriate. For example, department managers should be able to demonstrate that they collect and analyze data and, based on that data, develop and implement sound improvement plans, if needed.

The JCAHO does not want your PI plan to be a document that is simply dusted off and updated annually; your surveyors will question managers and leaders to ensure that they use the tool daily to help the hospital achieve its mission, vision, and strategic goals.

Evidence of compliance

Documentation

Your PI plan is one of the key PI documents surveyors will request to see. As they review it, they'll focus on identifying your hospital's approach to and methodology for PI. In addition, they'll ask to see multiple planning documents that pull together the full scope of the hospital's improvement and strategic planning processes (Figure 1.1). These strategic planning documents are key to the surveyors' ability to determine whether your hospital has taken its PI priorities seriously. They'll judge whether you've identified PI priorities and allocated appropriate resources to review the process, including money, time, and personnel. Those documents that show evidence of a process of prioritization and resource allocation will help demonstrate compliance with PI.1.

In addition, the following pieces of documentation will also help demonstrate your compliance with the PI.1 standards:

- **Mission and vision statements** provide surveyors with an overview of your values, services, and plans for the future. During the survey, surveyors will assess whether your PI process and priorities are in line with the hospital's values and services and whether they will contribute to the hospital's future direction.

- **Strategic planning documents** will help surveyors assess whether your institution considers PI priorities when appropriating resources.

- **The hospital's reporting structure** for monitoring PI activities helps surveyors understand how PI activities are prioritized, monitored, and reported.

- **Supporting minutes** from improvement teams or committees provide hard evidence that the PI process works. Minutes, reports, and results can also demonstrate that there is multidisciplinary participation in PI.

- **Documented results** of PI activities can include a list of current and planned measures (commonly referred to as *indicators*), process improvements, or results from the review of care processes for specific diagnoses.

The standards for documenting the participation of hospital leaders have changed. Previously scored in the PI chapter, the standards that refer to leadership's role in PI (PI.1 and PI.1.1) are now scored under LD.4.1 and LD.4.2. These standards require hospital leaders to participate in an active, collaborative, and interdisciplinary approach to PI. The wording of these standards has changed little, but their new placement indicates that the JCAHO expects leaders to demonstrate comprehension of, and a commitment to, your hospital's PI program.

Interviews

Leaders should expect to field the following types of questions during the chief executive officer/strategic planning and resource allocation interview, the leadership interview, the medical staff leadership interview, the nursing leadership interview and the hospital department director interview:

- Have you been educated and trained in the principles of PI?

- Do you use PI principles in your daily operations?

- Do you require your managers to develop, implement, and use quality plans in each area?

- Based on your strategic plan, what are the key processes in your hospital?

FIGURE 1.1

Demonstrating integration among strategic, operational, and quality planning

You should be able to demonstrate that the strategic plan for your hospital is directly linked to your major operating goals, and that these in turn drive key quality/performance improvement goals.

Strategic plan (excerpts)	Annual hospital goals (excerpts):	Performance improvement plans in relevant areas
	These might be found in hospital-wide planning documents, departmental goals, incentive compensation plans and performance reviews, or other documents.	*The hospital-wide quality plan will focus on a few key goals. Departmental or divisional or other more detailed plans will elaborate on those and other goals.*
We will improve the health of the communities we serve . . .	**Goal:** Conduct 75 screening sessions for common problems. **Goal:** Conduct early intervention programs for low-income pregnant teens.	**QI Plan:** Achieve targeted attendance and consumer satisfaction levels at these sessions. Conduct sample follow-up 6 months later to determine what percentage of individuals counseled to modify lifestyle or seek follow-up care did so. **QI Plan:** Achieve targeted attendance and consumer satisfaction levels at these programs. Achieve targeted birth weight and APGAR scores and demonstrate performance superior to a cohort that did not receive early intervention. Measure breast-feeding success rates at 6 months postpartum, compare to nonintervention cohort and national literature on breast-feeding in this population. Measure repeat pregnancies for 3 years.
We will contribute to the continuous improvement of medical care consistent with national guidelines and standards . . .	We will contribute to the improvement of medical care in our city . . . **Goal:** Implement clinical pathways with nationally accepted clinical practice guidelines for pediatric asthma admissions. **Goal:** Initiate an effort to reduce medication errors by 50% over the next 3 years.	**PI Plan:** Achieve targeted length of stay, repeat admissions, and successful outcomes for each hospitalization; measure asthma control through outpatient clinics at specified intervals to demonstrate improvement. **QI Plan:** Implement improved methods of collecting data on incidence of errors. Identify top three reasons for medication errors and enhance systems to prevent occurrence. Continue to encourage reporting and monitor improvement.

- What is your approach to PI?
- Do you have a written plan? When was the last time you looked at it?

Compliance tips

To ensure that your hospital complies with PI.1–PI.1.1, you should take the following steps:

1. Define and document a consistent, organization-wide approach to PI.
2. Discuss the hospital's PI plan and approach with your work force.
3. Focus on issues that matter to customers, such as decreasing wait times in one of your busy ambulatory areas or increasing the focus on patient education in one of your technologically advanced care centers.
4. Identify measurable characteristics of the organization, such as patient satisfaction or lengths of stay for specific diagnoses.
5. Involve all disciplines and areas of the organization, including the medical staff, in PI.
6. Integrate the hospital's PI plan with both hospital and departmental goals.
7. Verify that your PI philosophy has been successfully integrated into the hospital by reviewing the hospital's PI plan and past improvements.
8. Focus on flexibility—priorities can change quickly based on the market and internal organizational needs, so you should ensure that your plan can be easily adapted.

PI.2: Designing your performance improvement approach

JCAHO's requirements

To meet surveyors' expectations, you need to carefully define exactly how your hospital designs new processes or modifies existing ones. For example, as you work to refine a process or develop a new one, you should ensure that it is consistent with

- The mission and plans of the hospital
- The needs and expectations of key constituents
- The latest information and literature
- Sound business principles
- Baseline performance expectations

In other words, any time a hospital considers either changing a process or developing a new one (e.g., creating a new clinical service, upgrading the physical plant, or opening a subacute care unit) the organization should ask itself the following four questions to ensure that the JCAHO's standard PI.2 is met:

- Is this project consistent with the hospital's mission, values, and plans?
- Have we consulted our patients and employees to see if there is a need for this project and what their expectations for such a project would be?
- What do experts say about the design of such a project?
- What comparative data have we looked at to see if such a project has worked in other facilities?

The intent of this standard is not so much to control the growth and development of hospitals as it is to ensure that PI design criteria guide operational decision-making. Chapter 9 offers specific suggestions for complying with PI.2 standards in your hospital's business planning and PI frameworks.

What surveyors want

Surveyors will ensure that you do not develop new processes in a vacuum; they'll want to find evidence that you base your new initiatives on "customer" feedback, current clinical information and research, and sound business practices. They'll verify that you access clinical guidelines, reference databases, and benchmark information to compare your services to similar services provided by other organizations. Remember that you do not have to benchmark only against organizations of a similar size; sometimes you can learn a great deal by studying how smaller or larger organizations handle services akin to yours. For example, a large tertiary hospital might learn quite a bit by studying how a small hospital or nonhospital handles issues such as billing, reception, or confidentiality.

Surveyors will also check to see that your PI approach incorporates expectations for measurement and assessment based on your research and feedback. For example, an ideal PI approach would include the following steps:

1. Communication to obtain feedback about designing a new process or modifying an existing process
2. Assessment of feedback
3. Implementation of change
4. Measurement of change
5. Communication to obtain feedback on the results of the new or modified process

This cycle should continue until improvement is realized. Then, to make sure that improvement is sustained over time, the status of improvement should be monitored.

Your managers should also be able to demonstrate that they have a basic understanding of PI principles and methods. Once managers are clear on these concepts, leaders should determine what staffs' PI responsibilities are at every level. Basically, every employee should be oriented to your PI philosophy through discussions at regular staff meetings, employee newsletters, and participation in PI projects. By including the entire organization in your hospital's PI system, you'll integrate PI into the organization's daily operations and be able to demonstrate to surveyors that PI is a priority.

Evidence of compliance

Documentation

Documents, such as patient satisfaction survey results or minutes from community focus groups, will prove to surveyors that you carefully consider customer needs and work to improve existing processes. These documents should highlight your PI approach and outline exactly how your organization designs and redesigns its processes or services. In addition, the following documents will also be of key interest to surveyors as they gauge your compliance with the PI.2 standards:

- Your PI plan
- Strategic planning documents
- The hospital's reporting structure for PI information

- Supporting minutes of PI groups or committees, or both, demonstrating that the PI process works

- Customer feedback, including patient satisfaction results, community assessments, and internal employee satisfaction results to broaden your surveyors' understanding of your prioritization process

- Documentation showing how you design new services

- Documentation supporting clinical pathway development and implementation

Interviews

A critical part of every JCAHO is the set of interviews surveyors conduct with leaders and PI team members. See Chapter 4, Preparing for Survey, for a complete discussion. Participants in the PI coordinating group, PI team, and leadership interviews should be prepared to answer surveyors' questions on the hospital's approach to PI, such as the following:

- Do you have a prioritization method for multiple PI projects?

- Of the PI projects the hospital has completed to date, how important were the topics to patient care?

- How were the topics chosen? Who chose them?

- How did you choose the PI team members?

- Did these teams work on truly critical processes?

- Did these teams have access to ORYX and other comparative performance data as applicable to their project?

- Do the teams have concrete goals and time frames? Does the hospital's PI plan support these goals and time frames as well as promote flexibility?

Compliance tips

- It doesn't matter which PI methodology your hospital selects ("plan, do, check, act," "communicate, assess, implement, measure," or the "10-step model" are all acceptable PI models). It is most important that you use the chosen method consistently throughout your organization.

- Review all existing and new processes to ensure that they are consistent with the mission and vision of the organization. Ask yourself: "What is our mission? Do all the services we offer match that mission? Is there a gap that we have yet to fill?"

- Identify measurable characteristics of existing processes and new processes. For example, focus on issues that matter to your customers, such as reducing waiting times or speeding up the admissions and discharge processes.

- Gather the input of all appropriate disciplines and areas of the hospital when you design new processes or redesign existing processes, or both. Concentrate on determining who is responsible for each step in the process; these are the people who must be actively involved in your efforts to ensure that the new processes are efficient and effective.

- As you focus on creating new or updating old processes, be sure to integrate the new systems with departmental and hospital-wide goals. Always review your PI priorities in terms of the hospital's annual goals and objectives.

Chapter 1

- Focus on ensuring that your new processes are flexible; your organization should be able to quickly adapt to any changes it encounters down the road.

PI.3: Collecting and measuring data

JCAHO's requirements

Data collection is still one of the basic functions of a PI program. Only by systematically gathering data on a process or procedure can an organization objectively review its quality. The JCAHO requires that every hospital measure and collect data over time to gauge if improvements can be made in processes or outcomes.

In 1999, the JCAHO published standards that are less prescriptive when it comes to performance measurement. Monitoring of some indicators, once required, is now optional (Figures 1.2 and 1.3). You might be tempted to conclude that this change means you can eliminate many monitors and simplify your PI program. However, don't do so rashly.

Before eliminating any indicators, you should make a careful assessment of your monitoring program. You need to determine which measures are still required by other agencies or are important for reasons other than JCAHO compliance (see Figure 1.2). For example, you need to continue to monitor advance directives to remain compliant with the Health Care Financing Administration's Medicare Conditions of Participation. The sections that follow may help you to decide which optional indicators you can realistically stop monitoring.

What surveyors want

Surveyors want to find evidence that your hospital collects data on key processes and outcomes related to patient care and organizational processes. Because you may not have the time to collect data on every single process or procedure, you need to determine which issues are critical for your organization. With the PI.3 standards, the JCAHO intends to ensure that only relevant, useful, and important data are collected on vital aspects of care and service.

The processes you decide to evaluate will most likely still be centered around the JCAHO's 11 important patient functions listed in the *CAMH* (e.g., patient rights and organizational ethics, patient assessment, and care of the patient). It would be inadvisable for hospitals to discontinue measurement of patient-focused functions (assessment, treatment, education, patient rights, and continuum of care) or supporting functions (environment of care and human resources) that are now optional. This data is simply too vital to the monitoring of overall hospital performance. However, if you want to discontinue measurement in some areas, consider targeting your indicators for leadership, management, and governance, as some hospitals find it difficult to conceptualize measures for these functions.

The list of items to consider for measurement within your PI program has definitely become more explicit, and the list of required measures has decreased. However, it is important to note that the performance expectation is still inherent in the standards and should be based on the organization's mission, care and services provided, and particularly the population served. When reviewing the items to consider, focus on the following:

- **Appropriateness of admission and hospital stay** Although utilization management measures are now optional, they typically address such issues as nonacute days, length of stay, costs, and other indicators that are critical to demonstrating

FIGURE 1.2

Summary of required measures

Directions: Use this checklist to help you ensure that your hospital conducts measurements in each of the JCAHO-required areas. You must be able to prove to surveyors that you measure, assess, and improve (when appropriate) each of these areas. Remember, you must also measure all nine "dimensions of performance." (See Chapter 10 for more information on dimensions of performance.)

Required measure	In place?	Description of the measure	Notes
JCAHO functions			
Patient treatment: operative/invasive procedures			
• selection	❏Yes ❏No		
• preparation	❏Yes ❏No		
• performance	❏Yes ❏No		
• postprocedure care	❏Yes ❏No		
• patient education	❏Yes ❏No		
Patient treatment: blood administration			
• ordering	❏Yes ❏No		
• dispensing	❏Yes ❏No		
• administering	❏Yes ❏No		
• monitoring	❏Yes ❏No		
Patient treatment: medication administration			
• ordering	❏Yes ❏No		
• dispensing	❏Yes ❏No		
• administering	❏Yes ❏No		
• monitoring	❏Yes ❏No		
Patient treatment: restraint and seclusion (The JCAHO's TX chapter requires you to collect and monitor the use of restraint and seclusion by unit, shift, practitioner type, episodes per patient, and duration of use.)	❏Yes ❏No		
Patient satisfaction	❏Yes ❏No		
High-risk, high-volume, and/or problem-prone processes	❏Yes ❏No		
Newly designed or redesigned processes	❏Yes ❏No		
Outcomes related to resuscitation	❏Yes ❏No		
Requirements from other *CAMH* chapters:			
• infections (IC.2)	❏Yes ❏No		
• compctence (HR.4.3)	❏Yes ❏No		
• ongoing medical record review (IM.3.2.1)	❏Yes ❏No		
• information for patient care and operations (IM.8)	❏Yes ❏No		
• important processes (LD.4.3)	❏Yes ❏No		
• leaders' contributions (LD.4.5)	❏Yes ❏No		
• collection of information on environment of care (EC.1.3 – 1.9 and EC.3)	❏Yes ❏No		
Root-cause analysis of sentinel events	❏Yes ❏No		
Some type of measurement (generally using historical, comparative, or benchmark databases) to demonstrate a reduced risk of sentinel events	❏Yes ❏No		
Some type of measurement or documentation to demonstrate sustained improvement over time	❏Yes ❏No		

FIGURE 1.3

Considering measures for discontinuation

Directions: Use this checklist to help you decide whether to discontinue measurement in a particular area. Before discontinuing a measure, be certain to evaluate its importance carefully. Use the second part of this figure, "Issues to Consider Before Eliminating Performance Measures," to help you decide. You should consider other regulatory, professional, and legal monitoring requirements. As always, document fully any decision to discontinue measurement.

Measure to consider	Continue (C) or discontinue (D)	Required by other regulatory agency/other reasons? (specify)	Reasons to continue or discontinue
JCAHO functions			
Patient rights and organization ethics (RI)	❏C ❏D		
Assessment of patients (PE)	❏C ❏D		
Care of patients (TX) (See "Required measures," Figure 1.2)	❏C ❏D		
Patient and family education (PF)	❏C ❏D		
Continuum of care (CC)	❏C ❏D		
Improving organization performance (PI)	❏C ❏D		
Leadership (LD)	❏C ❏D		
Management of the environment of care (EC)	❏C ❏D		
Management of human resources (HR)	❏C ❏D		
Management of information (IM)	❏C ❏D		
Surveillance, prevention, and control of infection (IC)	❏C ❏D		
Other resources			
Performance measures related to accreditation and other requirements	❏C ❏D		
Risk management	❏C ❏D		
Utilization management	❏C ❏D		
Quality control	❏C ❏D		
Staff opinions and needs	❏C ❏D		
Behavior management procedures	❏C ❏D		
Outcomes of processes or services	❏C ❏D		
Autopsy results	❏C ❏D		
Performance measures from acceptable databases	❏C ❏D		
Customer demographics and diagnoses	❏C ❏D		
Financial data	❏C ❏D		
Infection control surveillance and reporting	❏C ❏D		
Research data	❏C ❏D		
Performance data identified in the functional chapters	❏C ❏D		
Appropriateness and effectiveness of pain management	❏C ❏D		
Outcomes of clinical practice guidelines	❏C ❏D		

FIGURE 1.3 (cont'd)

Issues to consider before eliminating performance measures

Have you monitored the measure for an appropriate length of time, using appropriate sampling methods?	❏Yes ❏No
Have you demonstrated that the measure shows that your hospital's performance was within an acceptable level, based on comparative data, past performance, or other benchmarks?	❏Yes ❏No
Have you evaluated the measure in light of your hospital's overall goals for quality improvement and demonstrated that it does not contribute significantly to accomplishing those goals?	❏Yes ❏No
Have you determined that the measure is not necessary for other accreditation or regulatory purposes (e.g., to satisfy the requirements outlined in one of the JCAHO functional chapters, or your state's Department of Public Health, Health Care Financing Administration, the Food and Drug Administration, the College of American Pathologists, etc.)?	❏Yes ❏No

appropriateness of care. In addition, these are measures that most hospitals need for business reasons. You might think twice before eliminating them.

- **Employee satisfaction and needs** Many hospitals gather feedback from employees via surveys and other vehicles, as most leaders recognize the importance of assessing and addressing work force concerns, and because it's important to involve workers who are closest to a process in improvement initiatives. So, if you have included "staff input and communication" as part of your PI program, you might want to continue this process.

- **Behavior management** This is defined by the JCAHO as the use of basic learning techniques, such as conditioning, biofeedback, reinforcement, or aversion therapy, to manage and improve human behavior. If used, these processes and patients' outcomes should be considered for measurement on a continuing basis and include assessment of the patients', families', and clinical staff's perceptions.

- **Risk management** Given JCAHO's focus on sentinel events and the national focus on medical errors, it is unlikely that any hospital would discontinue tracking risk management indicators at this time. You will want to ensure that they are well-targeted to your population, your historical areas of potential problems, and the JCAHO's current focus (their series of bulletins on sentinel events is available at www.jcaho.org/edu_pub/sealert/se_alert.html). In addition, your PI linkage to the risk management program should be sensitive enough to identify potential systems problems leading to incidents (or "near-miss" incidents), and should ensure prompt root cause analysis and systems improvement where indicated, including follow-up measurement.

- **Autopsy results** Considerable national attention has been paid to the issues of low autopsy rates and inattention to autopsy data. Autopsy results can be integrated into medical quality improvement as a feedback loop to clinicians. As a result, you might find your medical staff leaders urging you to retain autopsy indicators. You should carefully assess the value of these indicators before eliminating them.

- **Infection control data** The JCAHO standards on infection control still require hospitals to monitor, report, and make effective use of infection control data. Don't let the monitoring activity lapse because infection control is listed as an "optional" indicator in the PI chapter.

- **Quality control** Although the JCAHO no longer requires measurement of this function, other organizations still do. For example, the College of American Pathologists requires hospitals to monitor quality control (QC) indicators for laboratories; the Food and Drug Administration requires hospitals to monitor QC indicators for mammography and the pharmacy; and the American Association of Blood Banks requires hospitals to monitor QC indicators for blood services. You must also consider the requirements of your state department of public health. In addition, failing to monitor QC may void manufacturers' warranties on equipment and may leave your hospital vulnerable during lawsuits.

In 2000, the Joint Commission announced two new items to consider for measurement: (1) appropriateness and effectiveness of pain management, and (2) outcomes of clinical practice guidelines use.

Hospitals should focus on collecting data to monitor the stability of existing processes, identify opportunities for improvement, and identify changes that will lead to improvement and sustained improvement.

In addition, surveyors will ensure that you measure the specific processes and outcomes defined in standards PI.3.2 and PI.3.3 and their related substandards, including the following:

- **High-risk operative, other invasive, and noninvasive procedures** Review how well the hospital (1) selects these procedures, (2) prepares patients for them, (3) performs them, (4) monitors patients during these procedures, (5) cares for patients after them, and (6) educates patients and their families about them.

- **Medication use** Because virtually every patient in the hospital receives medication, you should consistently measure and monitor how well the hospital (1) prescribes or orders, (2) prepares and dispenses, (3) administers, and (4) monitors the effects of medication.

- **Blood use** Because the use of blood or blood components may pose an unnecessary risk to the patient, blood use performed in the hospital must be measured, including how well the hospital (1) orders, (2) distributes, (3) handles, (4) dispenses, (5) administers, and (6) monitors the effects of blood and blood components on patients.

- **Appropriateness of admissions and hospital stays** Review the appropriateness of admissions and hospital stays by collecting data, such as the ages, diagnoses, problems, and levels of care of patients, and comparing them over time to assess appropriateness, consistency of care, and appropriate utilization of resources.

- **Patient satisfaction** To ensure that your hospital provides appropriate services and has a high level of patient satisfaction, it must assess the needs and expectations of those it serves and gather feedback from patients.

- **Employee satisfaction** Like patient satisfaction, employee satisfaction also helps improve patient care. Does your organization conduct regularly scheduled meetings with staff to discuss performance and opportunities for improvement? Does your organization conduct employee satisfaction surveys or have an employee suggestion box? Evidence of these types of activities demonstrates compliance with this standard.

- **Behavior management** Monitor these processes and patients' outcomes on a continuing basis; include assessments of the patients', families', and clinical staff's perceptions.

- **Ongoing data collection and review** The hospital should conduct ongoing data collection and review of specific activities in the hospital, such as (1) autopsy results, (2) risk management activities, and (3) QC activities for specific areas such as clinical laboratory, diagnostic radiology, dietetic service, nuclear medicine, and radiation oncology.

Evidence of compliance

Documentation

Your primary evidence of compliance with the PI.3 standards will be the section of your PI plan describing your data collection and measurement process. In addition, you should ensure that your prioritization process is clearly described in the plan and that all the following documents are ready for surveyors' review:

- Results of ongoing data collection and reviews.

- Strategic planning documents, including feasibility studies related to new services.

- Supporting minutes from PI groups and committee meetings that highlight action taken as a result of the data gathered.

- An inventory of current measures or indicators used throughout the hospital and cross-referenced to the 11 JCAHO functions. (Although not required, this will be helpful to the surveyors in determining whether you evaluated and included key processes within your PI program.)

- Results of satisfaction surveys of patients, physicians, employees, and other customers used to assess specific PI projects.

- Description of departmental team and committee improvement initiatives resulting from the collection, measurement, and review of data.

- Results of reviews of invasive procedure, medication usage, blood utilization, utilization management, pathology, and risk management quality.

- Results of ORYX/core measures data tracking results.

In 2000, the JCAHO moved its discussion of ORYX and core performance measurement from the PI chapter to the Accreditation Participation Requirements chapter. This move shouldn't change your ORYX activities. For more specific information on the ORYX initiative and the introduction of core measures, see Chapter 3.

Interviews

Your surveyors will also gauge how well your organization measures and collects data during a number of interviews with leaders and staff. For example, in the leadership or PI interviews or patient unit visits, the surveyors may ask leaders and caregivers any of the following questions to help them get a sense of your data measurement and collection practices:

- Which of the JCAHO functions have you monitored through data collection of processes and outcomes?

Chapter 1

- Do you include process measurement as well as outcome measurement in your PI activities?
- What are some examples of measures you have recently implemented that were important to patients?
- Who collects your data?
- How is it collected?
- What happens once the data is collected?

Compliance tips

As you decide which processes or procedures to review for PI, keep in mind that JCAHO surveyors will want to see evidence that you focused on the required measures as indicated in Figure 1.2. In addition, they also want to see that you considered the "nonrequired" measures carefully before discontinuing them. The analysis criteria found in Figure 1.2 (p. 11) will help you decide what to do. These criteria and the discussion that follows will help your leaders expand their role in PI, thus helping your organization comply with LD.4.1 and LD.4.2. Ideally, you should document this assessment process by keeping minutes for all meetings. Or you might decide to make a formal report to your quality oversight committee: List each measure that you propose to discontinue and briefly address each of the points identified in Figure 1.2 to help justify your decisions.

To demonstrate a thorough review of your program, consider including a brief review of discontinued measures in an annual quality improvement program self-assessment. If the self-assessment reveals negative effects that resulted from the elimination of these data sets, you can revisit the decision to discontinue them. If it does not, you'll have further documented and justified the elimination process.

PI.4: Evaluating data

JCAHO's requirements

PI.4 and its substandards describe how you should evaluate and use collected data. For example, the JCAHO requires you to objectively review and improve new or existing processes by

- Collecting data in a systematic manner (PI.4)
- Utilizing statistical quality controls (PI.4.1)
- Trending data over time (PI.4.2)
- Intensively analyzing undesirable patterns or trends in performance and sentinel events (PI.4.3) (See Chapter 11 for a complete discussion of the sentinel event standards.)
- Utilizing data gathered to identify changes that will lead to improved performance and reduce the risk of sentinel events (PI.4.4)

What surveyors want

For several years, the JCAHO has been warning the field that assessment of collected data was relatively weak. Surveys have gone easy on this element of the standards, but JCAHO official publications have emphasized that thorough assessment, including the use of statistical analysis where appropriate, is expected and that this would be an area of increasing focus in the future.

How do you collect and measure data and information? What do you do when the data suggests that an area needs improvement? When do you implement a more intensive assessment of the information? How do you determine your key improvement priorities? These are the issues that are most important to surveyors when they judge your compliance with the PI.4 standards.

Every hospital must be able to prove to JCAHO surveyors that it measures and collects data related to its own important aspects of care. Surveyors are interested in seeing that hospitals select and prioritize PI objectives important to the people they serve.

Surveyors will also focus on how well you select and evaluate your improvement initiatives. You need to be able to demonstrate that you select your PI initiatives wisely and that you carefully evaluate processes that are important to patients and other customers for their efficacy, appropriateness, availability, timeliness, effectiveness, continuity, safety, and efficiency. Surveyors will check to see that you examine the quality of all the required measures as well as those organization-specific items that you have identified in your prioritization process. Examples of such items include

- Pre- and postoperative (including pathologic) diagnoses identifying a major discrepancy or a pattern, including those identified during specimen review
- Adverse events during anesthesia
- Reactions to blood transfusions
- Medication use
- Critical incident review and sentinel event analysis

You should be able to prove that you track the progress of your PI efforts and be able to demonstrate evidence of improvements.

In addition, in 1997 the JCAHO announced the ORYX initiative, which requires that hospitals collect standardized performance data and submit the results to the Joint Commission. In 1999, they announced the pending addition of core performance measures. You will need to ensure that you meet the ORYX and evolving core measure reporting requirements described in Chapter 3.

Evidence of compliance

Documentation

Meeting standards PI.4–PI.4.4 requires you to use aggregated, trended, and analyzed data to demonstrate measurable improvement in outcomes. Nothing less will suffice. Your primary evidence of compliance will be the outline of your evaluation process in your PI plan. Other documents such as these will help you prove to surveyors that you properly evaluate data:

- Documents indicating **ongoing data collection and reviews**.
- **Minutes from discussions with leaders** specifically highlighting the review of aggregated, trended, and analyzed data.
- **Supporting minutes of PI groups** or committees, or both, focusing on the actions taken as a results of the review of data.
- **Inventory of current measurements** within the hospital, highlighting measures relating to the JCAHO-defined functions.

- Documentation of **intensive assessment in response to the issues required by JCAHO** as well as others identified within your hospital, such as sentinel events, medication administration, or blood administration.
- Inventory of clinical performance measures as required by the JCAHO's **ORYX/core measures initiative**.

Interviews

Surveyors will also ask participants of the PI coordinating group interview a number of targeted data evaluation questions, including

- Who reviews PI data once it is collected?
- How is that review conducted?
- Do you look at historical data to see if improvements or unfavorable trends occurred over time?
- How do you know when a statistical variation points to a trend that needs to be addressed?
- Do you set expected completion times for your improvement teams?
- Has data ever pointed to a problem with an individual? If so, how did you respond?
- Do you stop collecting data when evidence suggests there are no issues?
- How have data collected through the ORYX process affected the PI program?

Compliance tips

- Over time, show evidence of measurement and data collection related to your organization's important processes. "Over time" is the key phrase. It is your organization's responsibility to prioritize and choose PI activities based on your identified needs, and over the 3 years between JCAHO surveys, you should easily be able to document measurement and sustained improvement. Surveyors are interested in seeing that hospitals select and prioritize performance measure objectives important to the people they serve as well as measuring those items that are required by the JCAHO and other regulatory agencies.

- To ensure that they meet both these standards and the needs of their customers, many hospitals first identify their PI objectives and then work to link the objectives back to one or more chapters of the *CAMH*. For example, if your hospital worked to improve the confidentiality and continuity of information gathered during the admissions, this initiative could potentially link to the following chapters of the *CAMH*: patient rights, assessment, leadership, PI, information management, and continuum of care. Because many of the chapters' requirements overlap, one PI initiative can easily link to three or more JCAHO functions.

- Use appropriate statistical techniques. Use control charts or other analytic tools to document data collection and comparisons. These documents can be used during a survey to show evidence of this activity.

- Use the most current literature, information from reference databases, and baseline performance expectations to compare internal and external comparisons of data and performance.

- Assess discrepancies in outcomes, sentinel events, adverse reactions, and individual competency issues. Offer staff members opportunities to improve their performance as well as improve upon the processes that are found to be inferior.

- Comply with all ORYX/core measures data collection and reporting requirements described in Chapter 3.

PI.5: Making improvements

JCAHO's requirements

PI.5 represents the culmination of all your work in complying with PI.1–PI.4. If you've planned and designed your PI system effectively and have measured and assessed all data according to JCAHO standards, you should have no trouble implementing improvements and demonstrating that your hospital has significantly bettered its performance (PI.5).

The JCAHO wants to see that you have taken all the information you gathered and assessed and used it to develop, test, and implement an improvement plan. If you should determine that a problem is the result of an individual's poor performance and that person refuses or is not able to improve, you must work to solve the problem, perhaps by revising his or her job description or modifying clinical privileges.

What surveyors want

How do you prove that you've made improvements? Surveyors will review the decision-making process for prioritizing and selecting improvement projects outlined in your PI plan and verify that you've followed those guidelines. They'll also check to see that you've considered the impact of any changes you made on patients, their families, physicians, and other hospital employees.

The hospital should be able to demonstrate that any changes made to a process or procedure were effective and implemented correctly. Surveyors will ensure that you monitored the performance of all new processes and conducted baseline monitoring to measure the performance of areas that are of key importance to patients, families, and other customers. Improvement teams should have a clear understanding of the hospital's PI process to develop and implement effective action plans. If an improvement wasn't completely successful, surveyors will check to see that you figured out what went wrong and then worked to correct the problem.

Evidence of compliance

Documentation

To give surveyors a clear understanding of your PI process, present the following documents in a single binder to show your compliance with the PI.5 standards:

- Your hospital's strategy on developing and implementing action plans for PI
- Sample actual action plans
- Sample documented results of these actions

Include customer surveys, comparisons with other providers, and charts describing the information flow to the governing board to provide a comprehensive picture of your PI program.

Chapter 1

Interviews

Participants in the PI coordinating group, PI team, and leadership interviews should also be prepared to answer surveyors' questions on improvements the hospital has made, such as the following:

- Have PI projects produced results that are affecting how the hospital is doing today?
- Did these projects meet your expectations?
- Are managers managing differently? Are managers in the learning mode daily?
- Are the key processes as described in your PI plan and the strategic plan getting better, worse, or staying the same? How do you know?
- Do your PI teams support both individual and work group improvement?

Compliance tips

To demonstrate that your hospital meets the PI.5 standards, offer your surveyors evidence of improvements related to the following:

- **Individual performance** This can be as simple as implementing safety education classes to improve fire drill response, or it can be specific to performance expectations for one job category.

- **Department performance** For example, many hospitals concentrate on reducing waiting times in ambulatory departments to improve patient satisfaction.

- **Hospital performance** By concentrating on improving hospital admissions, lengths of stays, and costs per patient, you can demonstrate an overall improvement in hospital financial performance. In addition, by focusing on improving the patient care process and streamlining services, you can also improve patient satisfaction.

- **Patient processes and outcomes** You can use process flow diagrams to show surveyors how you map out and redesign patient care processes and improve patient care outcomes.

- **Collaborative, multidisciplinary processes** Remember to include everyone along the continuum when you focus on improving a patient care process. For example, you might need to include the preadmission counselor, the admission clerk, caregivers (from nursing and respiratory to food and nutrition), discharge planners, and pastoral counselors. This approach will ensure a full look at the process and a more focused goal for improvement.

Chapter 2

Understanding Other Standards Related to Performance Improvement

After reading Chapter 1, you will find it evident that the performance improvement (PI) standards have the potential to affect activities and processes within individual departments as well as across your entire hospital. PI requirements are not found only in the PI standards. Many other standards in the *Comprehensive Accreditation Manual for Hospitals (CAMH)* are directly or indirectly related to PI. For example, the leadership (LD) standards describe exactly how leaders should manage all PI efforts, the human resources (HR) standards teach hospitals how to improve staff competency and staffing levels, and the information management (IM) standards require you to improve the quality of information in your organization. You need to integrate PI into every process or procedure in your hospital.

Read through this chapter to learn what you must do to meet these PI-related requirements. You'll learn what surveyors want to see, which supporting documents they'll review, what types of questions they may ask, and what you should do to ensure that your hospital's PI program is compliant.

JCAHO's patient-focused standards

JCAHO's requirements
In the eyes of the Joint Commission on the Accreditation of Healthcare Organizations (JCAHO) the top priority is patient care, and improving performance in all areas of care is critical to accreditation. You will find requirements to measure, assess, and improve processes and outcomes of patient care in several areas of *CAMH*: patient rights and organizational ethics (RI), assessment of patients (PE), care of patients (TX), patient and family education (PF), and the continuum of care (CC).

The PI standards require you to measure a number of specific processes by focusing your review efforts on some of the more high-risk patient care procedures. You are required to look for opportunities to improve areas such as operative and other invasive procedures, noninvasive procedures, medication and blood use, and patient satisfaction.

What surveyors want
The RI standards require you to advocate and maintain the rights of patients, their families, and your staff members, and to conduct your business ethically. You should be able to prove to surveyors that you work to measure and improve your processes for addressing patient satisfaction and ethical issues to help you better meet the needs of patients, their families,

and your staff. Many hospitals use a benchmarking approach to measure patient satisfaction and compare it to that of other organizations in their markets.

The PE and TX standards set guidelines for the patient care process, specifically patient assessment and treatment. For example, surveyors will want to know how you assess patients to determine which treatment is most appropriate for them. Once a patient assessment is completed, many hospitals use clinical pathways to help them improve their approaches to diagnosis or treatment of specified diseases, injuries, or conditions. These pathways, or treatment maps, help hospitals evaluate treatment results more objectively and reduce the likelihood of practitioner errors and inconsistencies. All positive outcomes related to clinical pathways, such as a consistency in length of stay per diagnosis and increased patient satisfaction, will be evidence of improvement for surveyors.

Surveyors also want to see that you comply with the PF standards by improving patient and family education. Shorter stays and technological advances in medication and treatment increase the need to make sure that patients understand their role in their own care. For example, patients' understanding of medication use and physical therapy techniques will increase the likelihood of a quick and full recovery. By educating your patients, you can improve their welfare and their satisfaction with your hospital.

Finally, to ensure that you meet the continuum of care standards and that you measure and improve the CC in your hospital, surveyors will review your admission and discharge planning processes. The assessment, reassessment, transfer, care, and discharge of a patient can be a monumental task, and one that can always stand improvement. Using patient satisfaction results to improve a portion of the continuum, developing and implementing clinical pathways, or focusing on the availability of post-hospital care are all examples of measuring and potentially improving the continuum. These processes are constantly scrutinized by patients, staff, physicians, and family members and could potentially generate successful PI projects.

Evidence of compliance

With the emergence of new standards regarding pain management, you have an opportunity to meet the whole range of PI and related standards embedded in these chapters on patient-focused functions while addressing a topic of significant importance to your patients. Consider selecting pain management or restraints (another topic of current focus for JCAHO and for federal regulators at the Health Care Financing Administration) as an integrated PI initiative, which will demonstrate your ability to bring interdisciplinary collaboration to a complex problem.

Interviews

Your PI efforts in these patient-focused areas may be surveyed during the following sessions:

- Patient and family education interview.
- Ethics interview.
- Visits to patient care units.
- Medication use and nutrition interview.
- Operative and other invasive procedures interview.
- The continuum of care interview.

Typical questions surveyors may ask include the following:

- How have your caregivers integrated patient and family education into care?
- How do you measure the effectiveness of your patient and family education program?
- Do you have an ethics committee? Does the committee protect patient rights and organizational ethics?
- What improvements have you made in the area of patient rights and organizational ethics during the last year?
- What PI activities have you participated in? How do they relate to the care process?
- What are the hospital's adverse drug reaction rates?
- How do you monitor medication use and administration?
- What improvements have you made in the areas of medication use and operative and other invasive procedure review?
- Have you focused on the admitting or discharge process within PI? Have you made improvements in the process based on input from your patients?

Documents

Surveyors may review any of the following documents to gauge your level of compliance with PI requirements, depending in part on which PI priorities you have selected:

- An **inventory of current measurements** within the hospital, such as patient satisfaction, staff satisfaction, or consistency in outcomes (particularly those related to clinical pathways).
- Results of patient, physician, employee, and other customer **satisfaction surveys**.
- Descriptions of **departmental and committee quality initiatives** within the care process.
- Results from **quality reviews** of the following key areas: operative and other invasive procedures; pharmacy and therapeutics, including medication administration; blood utilization; utilization management; autopsy results; and risk management.
- **Poster presentations** for PI activities related to patient-focused functions.

Compliance tips

Surveyors will explore whether you have truly improved performance in the areas that directly affect patient care. They will raise this topic with caregivers and leaders in the interview sessions mentioned above. Caregivers and leaders, including medical-staff leaders, should be prepared to discuss data gathered on issues of key interest to surveyors such as those affecting

- Important patient populations. (Familiarize yourself with the data the hospital has collected to evaluate high-risk, problem-prone, or high-profile procedures, gauge community needs, and evaluate strategic opportunities. For example, surveyors may want to see that you've evaluated the process for medication use, the speed of admissions, the length of hospital stays, and staff views on performance and opportunities for improvement.)
- A large percentage of the patient population.
- Risk management, patient satisfaction, infection control (IC), or sentinel events.

- Operative and other invasive procedures; noninvasive procedures; medication administration; use of blood/blood components; appropriateness of admissions/hospital stays; patient/employee satisfaction/input; behavior management; autopsy results; and specified quality control.

Leadership (LD)

JCAHO's requirements

In Chapter 1, you gained a basic understanding of the JCAHO's requirements for PI. You need to have a plan in place to identify patient care issues, correct problems, remove obstacles, and improve performance, which ultimately improves the patient care process. But to successfully implement such a PI program in your hospital, you must have a foundation of solid leadership. Without the support of your leaders, your PI program will not succeed.

In its LD chapter, the JCAHO lists a number of standards that require leaders to take an active role in the hospital's PI efforts. For example, they must

- Develop a prioritization process for improvements (LD.1.4).
- Understand PI approaches and methodologies (LD.4.1).
- Select a single approach to PI for the hospital (LD.4.2).
- Keep up-to-date on the status of PI efforts in the hospital (LD.3.4.1).
- Effectively allocate resources to all PI efforts (LD.4.4–LD.4.4.4).
- Analyze the effectiveness of PI efforts (LD.4.5).

Previously scored in the PI chapter, the standards that refer to leadership's role in PI (PI.1 and PI.1.1) are now scored under LD.4.1 and LD.4.2. These standards require hospital leaders to participate in an active, collaborative, and interdisciplinary approach to PI. The wording of these standards has changed little, but their new placement indicates that the JCAHO expects leaders to demonstrate comprehension of, and a commitment to, your hospital's PI program.

What surveyors want

First, surveyors expect leaders to demonstrate that they have established a clear PI planning process for the hospital. Planning is critical to the future success of an organization, and within their planning process leaders must define how the hospital will prioritize its PI initiatives.

For example, leaders should establish a method for changing or redirecting resources in the event of an unusual or important circumstance. An unplanned, steady rise in admissions within a certain specialty might warrant allocating some additional resources to a particular unit—specifically, additional caregivers, additional resources, and additional space. Or perhaps a steady decline in patient satisfaction related to a specific area of care would justify the implementation of a PI team.

Next, leaders must demonstrate to surveyors that they have a working knowledge of the different PI models (Chapter 8) and clearly understand how well each might work (or not work) in their organization. For example, they should be schooled on

- The old idea of quality assurance, or "quality by inspection," which is the process of searching for defects in a process after the damage has already been done.

- The origins of continuous PI.
- The basics of process re-engineering and how it affects PI.

After they have studied a number of PI approaches, leaders must select one to use in your hospital. The "shotgun" approach to PI, in which each department uses whichever method it likes, leads only to chaos; all departments and areas in a hospital must use the same PI approach. In the case of most hospitals, this means selecting the simplest method possible, such as the PDCA (*p*lan, *d*o, *c*heck, *a*ct) approach. This approach has only four steps that can be learned easily, and is the PI method most widely used in the industry. However, as long as you can demonstrate that the chosen approach is consistently applied across the organization and doesn't omit any essential elements, you'll meet surveyors' expectations.

Surveyors will also look to ensure that a reporting system is in place to keep leaders up-to-date on all multidisciplinary PI efforts throughout the hospital. This cross-organization communication is emphasized throughout the accreditation manual.

Your leaders, including physician leaders, should be able to prove to surveyors that they support all PI efforts in your hospital. For example, leaders should encourage personnel to participate in PI by offering training on the hospital's PI approach and should ensure that staff have time to participate in PI teams. In addition, they are responsible for verifying that all of the information systems and data management processes in the hospital are designed to help PI teams collect and analyze data.

Finally, surveyors want to see that leaders take the time to reflect on, analyze, and assess the effectiveness of their hospital's PI programs. For example, many organizations conduct annual reviews of their accomplishments, highlighting PI, productivity, and financial successes. This is an excellent format for reporting to your hospital's governing body and serves as essential background information for selecting priorities for future improvement plans.

Evidence of compliance

Interviews

Leaders should be prepared to discuss how they oversee PI throughout the organization. For example, surveyors may ask questions such as these:

- What is your PI philosophy, and how does it relate to your mission and vision?
- How are you trained in PI?
- How do you prioritize PI activities?
- Can you offer examples of PI projects that have had a positive impact on the patient care process?
- How do leaders collaborate on PI projects?
- Are you using PI principles and tools in your daily work?
- How do you involve employees in PI?

Documents

The documents in the following list will prove that you have a PI plan related to your mission, vision, and strategic plan. Ideally, these documents will provide the surveyors with an overview of your hospital's management structure, management philosophy, PI

Chapter 2

philosophy, and resource allocation relative to PI. Each of these elements is necessary in demonstrating compliance:

- A PI plan and methodology
- Mission and vision statements
- Strategic planning documents
- The results of community assessments
- A description of your reporting structure for PI information
- Supporting minutes from leadership, management, or other committees, including board minutes with evidence of PI reporting
- Documented training for managers and leaders on PI
- Your PI budget
- Documentation following one PI project from start to finish

Compliance tips

- Ensure that your leaders define a consistent, organization-wide approach to PI and describe it in a documented plan.
- Be able to demonstrate to your leaders that you have communicated this plan to staff. This can be highlighted in minutes of committees, management meetings, and other meeting minutes. It can also be shown in memos and newsletters to the general work force.
- Involve leaders in all disciplines and areas of the organization in PI. Your PI teams should include general hospital staff and representatives from senior management, nursing leadership, and medical staff (MS) leadership.
- Develop a list of operational changes that have been made based on the results of PI projects.

Environment of care (EC)

JCAHO's requirements

Look closely at the organization of the environment of care (EC) chapter in the *CAMH*; it's divided into four distinct sections that should be quite familiar by now (i.e., plan, design, assess, and improve). Although the EC standards may not be specifically linked to PI, they still emphasize the need to work consistently to improve the environment of your hospital. The EC chapter's Information Collection and Evaluation System in particular meets all of the expectations for substantive PI data management.

Many hospitals use committees or work groups (similar to PI teams) to assess and monitor the following seven elements required by the EC standards:

- Safety management
- Security management
- Hazardous materials and waste management
- Emergency preparedness
- Life safety management

- Medical equipment management
- Utility systems management

What surveyors want

Surveyors want to see evidence that the hospital

- Has plans in place to address the seven elements of safety
- Provides appropriate EC training
- Measures the staff's knowledge and performance

Hospital safety officers should develop performance measures for EC for each safety element. Once established, these measures can be used to determine whether the hospital is meeting its goals and expectations. But before they can create useful performance measures, safety officers must answer a few questions, such as:

- What level of measured performance would cause you to believe your expectations are being met?
- How often will you review and report this information to your safety committee and other quality committees?
- Where will you get the data?
- How often will you collect the data?
- To whom will you report this information?

Evidence of compliance
Interviews

During their tour of the hospital, surveyors may ask staff how they have worked to improve the environment of the hospital; for example:

- How has the hospital worked to improve the fire alarm response rate in your area?
- How have you worked to improve your understanding of utility management?
- How have you improved your understanding of, and response to, disaster drills?

Documents

To meet surveyors' expectations for PI in the EC, safety officers must develop management plans for each of the seven key EC areas and implement appropriate performance measures across your organization. They must document the hospital's improvement efforts within each of these seven areas to demonstrate that the hospital consistently works to measure, assess, and improve the quality of its environment.

In addition, safety management committee and subcommittee meeting minutes can be used to demonstrate compliance with the standards. These minutes should coincide with the goals and objectives of the hospital's management plan and highlight actions taken to improve the environment within the seven areas as defined by JCAHO.

Compliance tips

- Develop plans that are consistent with the hospital's methods for assessment of the EC. For example, if the life safety management plan states that your staff must be knowledgeable about fire procedures, the hospital must have a mechanism in place to measure this knowledge.

- Use these plans to monitor and improve the EC by defining, assessing, and improving all safety elements when necessary.

- Document activities related to the assessment, monitoring, and improvement of the EC. Be prepared to share and highlight this information during survey. The PI activities can be documented in minutes, reports, and so on.

Human resources (HR)

JCAHO's requirements

A hospital cannot meet the needs of its patients if it doesn't have a competent, skilled work force. How does your organization ensure that an appropriate number of qualified, well-trained staff members are on duty at all times? Your HR department is responsible for continuously monitoring staffing levels and staff competency to ensure that patients receive only the highest quality of care (HR.3), and the only way they can meet this requirement is to consistently look for opportunities for improvement.

What surveyors want

Surveyors will judge how well the HR process for evaluating the competency of staff improves the quality of patient care. They will want to see evidence that the HR department has established clear job descriptions and initial staff qualifications for those jobs. In addition, they will want to review the performance evaluation process and specifically look at competency requirements, objectives, and results. Surveyors will look for consistency and a link from job description to performance evaluation to competency requirements. A single format for job descriptions and performance evaluations, though not required, will present an organized, cohesive image to the survey team.

Evidence of compliance

Interviews

PI will be discussed during the HR interview, and surveyors may ask questions such as these:

- What is the process for identifying, prioritizing, and improving staff education needs?
- How do you know you have enough staff?
- How do you know you have fully competent staff for their current responsibilities?
- What opportunities do you offer staff for self-improvement?

The competency assessment process review will also provide an opportunity to discuss PI. The focus during this session will be on individual employees. For example, if an individual had performance problems but was not willing to change, surveyors will want to know how you solved the problem.

Documents

The following documents relate to the process of hiring, training, monitoring, and retaining competent employees. By using these documents to show surveyors a snapshot of your HR process, they can better understand what your HR department has done to ensure that staff are competent and are working to improve their performance. These key documents include

- Explanations of your job description development, orientation, and performance evaluation processes.
- Documentation of employee recognition activities.
- Staffing and development information, including employee satisfaction surveys, course evaluations, and documented staffing levels.

Compliance tips

- Develop and implement processes that will help the hospital monitor and improve staffing levels, staff competency, and employee and patient satisfaction. Remember that this does not always mean adding more staff. It could be a plan to enhance flexibility in staffing. For example, job descriptions, employee orientation and education programs, and performance evaluations all will help outline the process the hospital has implemented to ensure the competence and improved performance of staff.

- Document all improvement efforts and be prepared to discuss them with surveyors. For example, the improvement efforts related to individuals will be discussed during the competence review session. How did you identify an individual's performance problems? What steps did you take to improve his/her performance? What role did the employee play in this process? Be prepared to give actual examples of success stories.

Information management (IM)

JCAHO's requirements

Information is an integral part of a healthcare organization's PI efforts. To deliver appropriate care to patients and monitor and improve that care, you need key information, such as patient-specific data included in the medical record, aggregate data used to support clinical and management decisions, and comparative data to support care decisions and planning.

What surveyors want

Although the main thrust of the *CAMH* IM chapter is to guide the capture, management, and use of information to potentially improve patient care and the infrastructure that supports patient care, a number of IM standards are focused on PI. They require the IM department to plan and design a system to gather supporting PI information, such as

- Accurate and timely patient-specific data to improve care decisions
- Pertinent aggregate and comparative data to improve processes related to patient care
- Current knowledge-based information that highlights state-of-the-art technology to enable the research and development of new patient care initiatives

The hospital must also demonstrate that it consistently works to benchmark its performance against that of similar organizations, such as hospitals within your network or system or hospitals of the same size and patient population. Therefore, the hospital must have a well-designed IM system that captures, reviews, and compares key pieces of data using standardized data sets, definitions, codes, classifications, and terms used throughout the hospital (IM.3.1.1). Only with these elements in place will the IM department be able to compare internal and external processes and determine where improvements must be made.

The hospital must have a strong system for integrating and retaining information (IM.6) to adequately support and improve the patient care process. All information systems, whether

Chapter 2

computerized or manual, must be compatible and linkable when necessary. This linkage is essential for maintaining and improving patient care. By providing a full view of the information, whether it is related to the patient care process or the management structure, care providers throughout your organization will have the ability to make informed decisions about which areas need improvement.

The medical record department must also work to improve the medical record by gauging the clinical pertinence of your records by measuring their accuracy, completeness, and timeliness (IM.3.2.1). The medical record is a key piece of information in your hospital, and its quality must be continuously reviewed to ensure that it meets all the requirements in IM.7.

Evidence of compliance

Interviews
The IM interview gives surveyors a chance to discuss the hospital's IM plan, how it was developed, your process for communicating information consistently and accurately, and how the hospital has worked to improve these functions. Questions surveyors are likely to ask include:

- What is your method for integrating data across the organization?
- What PI activities currently under way relate to IM?
- What comparative databases do you use in patient care PI activities?

Documents
Surveyors may request any of the following documentation to gauge whether the hospital is compliant with the IM standards:

- Meeting minutes, reports, and plans proving that your hospital assesses its information needs and that it works to meet those needs
- Policies and procedures reflecting your standards for uniform data definitions
- Policies and procedures that outline medical record content requirements
- Minutes or reports proving that the hospital conducts quarterly multidisciplinary medical record reviews designed to improve the quality of patient care information and to record completion rates
- An inventory and explanation of comparative databases your hospital uses in all PI efforts
- Evidence of steps taken to correct medical record delinquencies, if any

Compliance tips

- Educate leaders and other key individuals who collect, generate, and utilize data on the basics of IM so they are prepared to use and manage information effectively and efficiently.
- Assess and document both your internal and external information needs. This is critical to PI. To begin any PI project, you need information.
- Concentrate on improving the content, completeness, and accuracy of medical records through a thorough clinical pertinence review.
- Document activities related to the assessment, monitoring, and improvement of the IM processes.

Surveillance, prevention, and control of infection (IC)

JCAHO's requirements

The surveillance, prevention, and control of infection standards are designed to help you monitor, prevent, control, and reduce the risk of infection in your organization, and the best way to ensure that your hospital is compliant is to integrate IC into your hospital-wide PI process. You need a clearly defined system to gather data and other information on IC in your hospital and use it to prevent, reduce, and control infection.

In addition, standard IC.6 requires hospitals to prevent the transmission of infections from patients to staff. For example, your IC department should conduct activities to reduce nosocomial infection rates and hold inservices or other programs to teach staff and leaders about infection prevention.

What surveyors want

Surveyors need to understand how data is collected, communicated, and used to improve patient care. As with the *CAMH* EC chapter, you'll find that the data management skills defined in PI standards are completely applicable here. Surveyors will be interested in the number and qualifications of the IC staff, how the competency of IC staff is measured, and how hospital staff are educated and trained in IC.

Evidence of compliance

Interviews

Your IC coordinator will be expected to discuss the hospital's IC program and improvement initiatives with the surveyors. He or she should be prepared to answer questions such as these:

- What is the structure for surveillance and reporting of IC data and information?
- How are the data and information gathered used to improve patient care?
- How do you connect and integrate your IC program with your PI activities?

Documents

In addition, documents that demonstrate how you measure, assess, and improve IC should be available to surveyors. For example, the IC coordinator should prepare

- Policies and procedures defining your IC program and key issues that are important to your patient population and community, such as education about the prevention of tuberculosis or sexually transmitted diseases
- Reports and meeting minutes describing the results of IC improvement activities
- Improvement action plans describing how the hospital has worked to prevent and control nosocomial infections
- Documents demonstrating your use of comparative databases, if any, for setting targets for improvement

Compliance tips

- Ensure that your hospital-wide PI plan focuses on assessing and monitoring IC surveillance, prevention, and control activities.

Chapter 2

- Develop, implement, and document processes to measure, assess, and improve issues related to IC.

- Make sure that you have at least one ongoing PI activity aimed at infection prevention, and document it in meeting minutes, policies and procedures, and the IC scope of services.

Medical staff (MS)

JCAHO's requirements

As with any other member of your hospital, physicians must be involved in PI. Medical staff leaders are responsible for working collaboratively to implement and direct the ongoing assessment and improvement of patient care quality in your organization and carry out various PI-related responsibilities outlined in their bylaws, rules, and regulations. For example, the JCAHO requires the medical staff to continuously look for opportunities to improve the quality of care they provide (MS.4.2.1.12) in areas such as

- Medical assessment and treatment of patients (MS.8.1.1)
- Medication use (MS.8.1.2)
- Blood use (MS.8.1.3)
- Operative and other procedures (MS.8.1.4)
- Efficiency of clinical practice patterns (MS.8.1.5)
- Significant departure from established clinical practice patterns (MS.8.1.6)

The medical staff must also work to improve the following processes for and outcomes of patient care (MS.8.2):

- Patient and family education (MS.8.2.1)
- Coordination of care with other caregivers and hospital staff (MS.8.2.2)
- The accuracy, timeliness, and legibility of patient records (MS.8.2.3)

Again, this highlights the need for a multidisciplinary PI plan and a multidisciplinary view of the patient care process.

What surveyors want

Without the medical staff's cooperation, you cannot substantially improve patient care in your hospital. For example, surveyors will want to see that physicians are able to describe the PI process, how they participate in it, and how they educate themselves about new PI approaches and methods. Medical staff leaders should also understand how PI initiatives are identified and prioritized.

Evidence of compliance

Interviews

Surveyors will quickly discover whether your physicians actively participate in PI during interview sessions. Therefore, you should ensure that your physicians can describe their role in PI, including how they measure, assess, and improve both clinical and nonclinical processes and how they relate the results of these activities to patient care. For example, they should be prepared to respond to such questions as these:

- What is the hospital's PI model?
- Who is the PI coordinator, expert, or leader in your department?
- What is your role in the department PI program?
- How do you identify opportunities to improve patient care?
- What high-volume, high-risk, and problem-prone procedures do you perform?
- How would you get a PI project started?
- Who would collect data?
- What is your role in drug usage, blood usage, and surgical case reviews?
- What types of improvements have you made to patient care in the last year?
- How do you know improvement actually occurred and was sustained?
- How do you link PI information with individual clinical privileges? How do you compare practice patterns among privileged staff?
- How do you integrate comparative data from outside your hospital in assessing performance?
- Have you implemented clinical pathways that would highlight established clinical practice, integrate clinical guidelines, or reflect a study of comparative data?
- How do you evaluate individuals whose practice patterns are identified as being outside the norm as a result of measurement and assessment activities?

Documents

Documents that will demonstrate physicians' compliance with JCAHO PI requirements include

- References to clinical PI requirements in your hospital-wide PI plan
- A list of physicians who are members of PI committees
- Policies and procedures outlining the appointment and reappointment process for physicians
- A written description of how PI activities are integrated into clinical performance evaluations
- Reports and meeting minutes highlighting discussions and actions related to clinical PI activities
- Documents describing physician participation on improvement or clinical path teams
- Physician newsletter or other means of communicating PI information to staff

Compliance tips

- Ensure that requirements for clinical PI are defined in the hospital's PI plan.
- Demonstrate that the PI plan has been communicated to the medical staff.
- Integrate PI initiatives with all other goals of the medical staff and the hospital. For example, conduct an annual review of the PI plan and accomplishments with the physicians, perhaps during your annual review of management goals and objectives, to ensure that your focus is on improving performance and ultimately improving patient care.

Chapter 2

- Pull out the key standards in the *CAMH* that are important to the medical staff and explain them to physicians so that their direct involvement in the improvement of patient care is clear.

- Never inform physicians that they need to participate in PI simply because the JCAHO requires it. Instead, explain that their involvement in clinical PI projects will help their peers and other ancillary providers, as well as their patients.

- Don't coax or coddle difficult, recalcitrant, or disruptive physicians. Instead, ask a few good physician leaders (e.g., those who are liked and respected) how the hospital should appeal to these individuals.

- Make physician participation in PI a continuous and gradual process. Don't ask them for their undivided attention and time just before survey. Instead, take advantage of all teaching opportunities to spread your message. Use the existing forums, such as medical staff meetings, the staff newsletter, or materials passed out on appointment or reappointment, to teach physicians about PI over time.

- Work patiently with physicians. Deliver your clear message over and over again, always highlighting that it is important to patient care. If you say it the right way, with enough respect, physicians will pay attention.

- If the PI program has real substance and a contribution to make in improving patient care, there will usually be no shortage of physicians willing to work with you. The key hurdle is demonstrating this level of substance.

Governance (GO), management (MA), and nursing (NR)

JCAHO's requirements

Your hospital's governing board, senior managers, and nurse executives are just as responsible for complying with PI requirements as any other member of the hospital. For example:

- The governing body should direct and support PI within your hospital (GO.2.4 and GO.2.5).

- Senior managers, such as the chief executive officer (CEO), should ensure that PI initiatives are implemented according to the governing body's directions (LD.4.3 and LD.4.4).

- Nurse executives should implement mechanisms for assessing and improving care (NR.2–NR.4).

What surveyors want

The governing board should be able to demonstrate to surveyors that it

- Is involved in strategic planning

- Monitors the hospital's progress toward its mission and strategic objectives

- Carefully reviews all quality reports, including data of MS performance

- Supports all PI efforts and ensures that the hospital offers a single level of care to its patients

- Monitors the performance of the annual budget and approves targets for debt, liquidity, return on investment, profitability, and other important measures of financial performance

- Monitors the performance of new programs and joint ventures

- Evaluates the CEO's performance annually using specified targets
- Evaluates its own performance

Surveyors will be interested in how senior managers, such as your CEO, improve administration management. For example, they'll want to discuss any efforts that have been made to improve

- Operations
- Information and support systems
- Recruitment and retention of competent staff
- Conservation of physical and financial assets

Nurse executives should be prepared to discuss their PI efforts with surveyors in sessions such as the nursing leadership interview and visits to patient care settings. They should emphasize how they implement programs to measure, assess, and improve the quality of nursing care offered to patients. (Note that this must encompass all nursing care, regardless of the specific organizational structure in your hospital and regardless of whether some nurses report to a chain of command outside the nurse executive's own.) In addition, they should describe the organization's PI approach and feel comfortable discussing other PI issues, such as how they

- Implement multidisciplinary PI efforts
- Prioritize PI efforts
- Collect and assess data on new and existing processes
- Determine when more intensive assessments are required
- Design and implement PI initiatives

Evidence of compliance
Interviews

The governing board, senior managers, and the nurse executive can expect to discuss the hospital's PI efforts during interview sessions such as the CEO/strategic planning and resource allocation, leadership, MS leadership, NR leadership, and hospital department director's interviews. They should be prepared to answer questions on

- Their role in PI
- The method by which they were educated in PI
- How PI is integrated into the care process
- How PI activities have improved care in the hospital
- Staff training and hospital-wide support for PI
- How they individually lead PI within their scope of responsibility

Documents

Documents such as the following will all demonstrate compliance with these requirements:

- The hospital's PI plan
- Meeting minutes and reports highlighting discussions and actions related to clinical and nonclinical PI activities

Compliance tips

- Define a consistent, organization-wide approach to PI and review it with the governing board, senior leaders, and nurse executives in your organization. A comprehensive program must protect the basic level of patient safety, effectively identify processes or individuals with quality problems, and continuously scan for opportunities for improvement.

- Leaders should recognize and promote the fact that PI is a critical part of daily operations and must not be viewed as a separate task.

- Within the PI process and beyond, leaders should promote and encourage constructive, collegial, and collaborative relationships to improve patient care and the patient care environment.

Chapter 3

The ORYX Initiative and Core Performance Measures: New Challenges for Your Hospital

In 1996, the Joint Commission on Accreditation of Healthcare Organizations (JCAHO) announced that it would require hospitals to collect and submit standardized performance data to the commission. In 1997, the details of this new policy were finalized and published under the name ORYX. This initiative has potentially significant financial, accreditation, public relations, and marketing implications for every hospital. In this chapter, we examine the initial goals of ORYX, the problems associated with its implementation, how it has changed, and the introduction of the Core Performance Measure initiative.

What is ORYX?

The JCAHO details its ORYX program in the Accreditation Participation Requirements chapter of the *Comprehensive Accreditation Manual for Hospitals*. The initial goals of the ORYX initiative required all hospitals to select relevant measures from a preselected universe of test measures meeting JCAHO criteria. The Joint Commission would then collect the data directly from the measurement system on a quarterly basis. The data collection included a phased implementation plan covering a gradually increasing proportion of the hospital's population (ultimately requiring six measures as of January 1, 2000). Failure to comply with these requirements resulted in a special Type I recommendation with a follow-up response required; continued failure to comply would result in loss of accreditation.

However, the Joint Commission has changed course somewhat. As of 2000, the JCAHO has confirmed that ORYX will be completely replaced by the Core Performance Measure initiative in approximately 2002. Assessing core measures is JCAHO's attempt to collect data that allow for comparisons between hospitals and for the establishment of industry-wide quality benchmarks. ORYX should now be considered simply a "dry run" of the process of collecting and submitting standardized measures. It is unlikely that the JCAHO will do very much meaningful monitoring or intervention on the basis of ORYX data in the interim period before the Core Performance Measures replace them in approximately 2002.

Participating in ORYX

The JCAHO's standards have always required hospitals to participate in comparative performance improvement (PI), but the ORYX initiative took that requirement a step further. It required hospitals to make comparisons on issues that affect a substantial patient population. Ideally, this requirement was supposed to help hospitals focus on issues that matter to patients. In the short term, JCAHO surveyors will expect you to demonstrate that participation in the ORYX program has been integrated with PI to enhance the quality of patient care in your hospital. In the future, however, the JCAHO will hold hospitals to a much higher standard for accountability to a common set of performance measures, the Core Performance Measures.

From a practical point of view, the necessity of participation in ORYX and the core measures initiative is simply to maintain your accreditation status. It is not an option to decline to participate, as the program is established as a condition of continued accreditation.

Challenges of ORYX and the core measures

The most obvious challenge associated with ORYX compliance is a financial one. It takes time and money for you to select and implement (or change) a performance measurement system. Even if you are already using a JCAHO-approved system, you would be wise to look at it closely and verify that it is indeed the best one for your hospital to use. See Figures 3.1 and 3.2 for checklists that will help you decide which measurement system is most appropriate for your hospital.

The core measures initiative also presents other risks to your hospital. For example, the results of your measures will alert the JCAHO to problems in your organization. Although the Joint Commission has stated that it will not form judgments about a hospital based on these data, it has said that the data you submit will be monitored quarterly "to raise questions about" your organization's performance. In response to a noted problem, the JCAHO may contact your hospital to ask how apparent problems in the data have been addressed, or it may require a written progress report or on-site survey. Another possibly serious consequence of this process is that the JCAHO might allow the problematic data to become public at some point. Although the JCAHO does not plan to do so in the immediate future, its policy statement indicates that it might.

Thus, in theory, there could be public disclosure of your trended information. Also, as managed care organizations focus more heavily on securing quality information from your hospital, it is likely that they will begin to ask for the same performance information you provide to the JCAHO, as much as they now ask for a copy of your hospital's latest JCAHO survey report. You may decide not to honor such a request, but you may want to be in a position to assent to it with data that you know to be reflective of a high level of performance.

These data represent a significant source of risk to the hospital. It is important to select measures that are reliable, valid, genuinely helpful to the hospital in focusing on performance, and that reflect competent performance over time.

Selecting a performance measurement system

To participate in the ORYX/core measures program, you must select a performance measurement system approved by the Joint Commission. Each of the performance measurement systems participating in the ORYX/core measures program was selected by a national panel of experts according to a defined set of JCAHO-approved criteria. The

FIGURE 3.1

Making the first cut: which vendors' systems should you evaluate?

As you review the long list of ORYX-approved measurement systems you may feel intimidated. But it is fairly easy to make the first cut and determine which systems are truly appropriate for your hospital. Simply review each system and ask yourself

- "Do we have a good existing relationship with any of the ORYX-approved system vendors even if we're not using the ORYX-approved system at this time?" If so, you should strongly consider using one of the systems from a known vendor.

- "Do we have ongoing comparative analysis already in place in any of the areas covered by ORYX system vendors?" If so, you might choose to continue your comparative data collection plans and simply switch to an ORYX-approved system.

- "What are our top PI priorities this year, and which ORYX-approved vendors have systems that would help us measure these areas? Any vendor whose measurement systems match your hospital's PI priorities would be a logical choice.

Joint Commission provides a current list of performance measurement systems at this address: http://www.jcaho.org/perfmeas/steps/systems.html.

The JCAHO's position on the approved systems is somewhat curious. It notes that all systems in the approved list meet its screening criteria, but it still holds you accountable for determining how well the systems meet the criteria. Therefore, before you select a system, the JCAHO requires you to ensure that your approved performance measurement system

- Includes clinical, satisfaction, health status, and/or administrative/financial measures
- Is not exclusively based on individual performance
- Is related to an accreditation program (i.e., a hospital accreditation program)
- Includes an operational, ongoing, automated database that can identify each hospital and electronically transmit data for that hospital and the comparative database to the JCAHO
- Maintains data quality and accuracy
- Offers risk adjustment or explains why it cannot be done currently
- Offers each participating hospital annual comparative feedback on its performance
- Teaches each hospital how to use the comparative data
- Is useful and relevant for accreditation

Selecting measures for ORYX/core measures compliance

Once you've selected a performance measurement system, you must decide which measures your hospital should use. As you make your decision, you should focus on

- Selecting meaningful measures
- Avoiding unnecessary work
- Minimizing cost

Chapter 3

FIGURE 3.2

Evaluating your short list: choosing the one performance measurement system that's right for you

After you've selected your short list of top performance measurement systems, you need to take a close look at each of your candidates. In most cases, a small staff group will perform these system reviews. As much as possible, they should try to quantify their conclusions by ranking each system's performance for each of the criteria listed in the following chart on a scale of 1–3.

Simply scoring each system will give you a good sense of which is the best system for you. However, you should remember that not all criteria will be of equal importance to your hospital, and the quality oversight committee should rank which criteria are most important. Multiply the System Ranking score by that for Importance to Hospital to obtain an overall score. The lowest scoring items will best fit your needs.

Use the chart below to help you evaluate your "short list" of potential performance measurement systems.

Name of Measurement System _____

Criterion	Considerations to evaluate and document	System ranking 1 = perfect 2 = acceptable 3 = inferior	Importance to hospital 1 = essential 2 = valuable 3 = nice to have	Overall score	Notes
Are the measures in this system relevant to our patients?	What proportion of our patients or other services would be affected by these measures? How does this system reflect an important aspect of care and service?	1 2 3	1 2 3		
Are the measures in this system relevant to our PI goals for the year?	Which PI goals this year would the measures support?	1 2 3	1 2 3		
Are the measures practically focused? Are they measuring items we would change or improve if we found that our performance is not as good as we would like?	What processes will be evaluated by this measure? For example, if we are measuring cost of care, will we be measuring important issues like physician ordering, cost of supplies and inputs, and the efficiency of production of services?	1 2 3	1 2 3		

40 — Performance Improvement: Winning Strategies for Quality and JCAHO Compliance, Second Edition

FIGURE 3.2 (cont'd)

Do we have an adequate number of patients to obtain reliable findings on these measures?	What number of patients do we expect to have available? For instance, if this is measured through a survey, what response rate do we expect? If it is measured through chart review, what sample sizes will we need to abstract?	1 2 3		1 2 3
Are the potential costs reasonable in light of the expected benefit?	Define what it will cost to acquire, implement, and maintain the system, considering both direct and indirect costs.	1 2 3		1 2 3
What is the technical feasibility of using this system?	Consider the hardware and software compatibility issues of each candidate vendor system. If our hospital cannot communicate with the vendor's computer in the manner required, then the system is not feasible and further review is not warranted. On the other hand, often compatibility is a matter of cost, and we may find that we can use the system but do not choose to do so due to excessive costs for the projected benefits.	1 2 3		1 2 3
Are the data elements of each measure defined clearly and consistently? Is the underlying process described accurately?	Review vendor claims, other hospital users' feedback about the system, and specific data collection and analysis algorithms to help determine whether the system will meet our needs.	1 2 3		1 2 3
Does the measurement system meet all of the JCAHO's requirements?	Briefly summarize how the measure fulfills the JCAHO requirements. The vendor should be able to provide its perspective on this issue and be able to comment on future criteria and its plans to meet those criteria.	1 2 3		1 2 3
Are the measures of interest to management and clinical leadership? (E.g., if it's not already on our PI plan for the year, there is interest in adding it to the plan.)	All medical and clinical leaders should agree on which system to use and be willing to use its measures and act on all findings.	1 2 3		1 2 3

Chapter 3

Focusing on meaningful measures

The JCAHO expects your hospital to demonstrate (usually through committee meeting minutes) that the measures you select are meaningful for the types of patients you serve and are consistent with your PI goals for the year. This will require you to formally evaluate your candidate systems according to the JCAHO's selection criteria and outline your own hospital's priorities and requirements to refine your choice further.

The JCAHO recommends that you set up a formal evaluation and selection process using predefined criteria and priority matrices. However, it is essential that you be able to demonstrate through your leadership process (again, most likely through quality oversight committee, medical executive committee, and/or board committee minutes) that you have evaluated

- The relevance of a measure to your patients (i.e., "This is something that we have reason to believe will be important.")
- The relevance of this measure to your PI goals for the year ("This is something we know we want to work on.")
- Whether the focus of the measure is practical ("This is something we can change or improve if we find that our performance is not as good as we would like.")
- Whether you will have an adequate number of patients available to obtain reliable findings
- Whether the expected costs are reasonable in light of the expected benefit
- Whether the system is technically feasible for you to use
- Whether the measure itself has face and content validity (data elements are defined clearly and consistently and the measure describes an underlying process accurately)
- Whether the measure comprehensively fulfills the JCAHO criteria
- Whether the measure is of interest to management and clinical leadership ("If it's not already on our PI plan for the year, is there interest in adding it to the plan?")

Avoiding unnecessary work

As you work to comply with the JCAHO's ORYX requirements, try to avoid redundant or unnecessary work and ensure that your selected ORYX indicators also meet other needs in the hospital, such as those for meaningful performance data comparisons and compliance with the required JCAHO PI measures (see Chapter 10).

Therefore, as you inventory your PI measures each year, you should ensure that all of your selected ORYX measures are part of the inventory and thus are part of your total compliance with PI.3 (measurement). This avoids duplicate or unnecessary work. Also, if you are already using an approved measure from one of the JCAHO's selected PI measurement systems in your general PI program, consider whether you should register it as one of your ORYX-compliance measures.

You may also find that information systems vendors with whom you have an existing relationship are now broadening their product line to meet the JCAHO's requirements. If they offer a measurement system that is approved by JCAHO and that requires no new data collection, you will want to evaluate such opportunities early on.

Minimizing cost

Finally, you should always ensure that your selected measures are cost-efficient to implement. For example, before you choose a measure, consider the costs of

- Participating in the comparative system (i.e., "What fees or computer hardware/software will be required?")
- Collecting the data on the measures ("Do we have the human and computer resources needed to collect this data?")
- Analyzing and assessing the data as they are produced
- Investing energy in a new area of focus and moving resources from other priorities already in place
- Potential exposure to the hospital if the data demonstrate an unfavorable trend or variance
- Potential investment in process improvement if the measure reveals poor performance (this cost would of course be offset by the ensuing benefits in patient care or other operational improvements)

More information on ORYX

If you have any questions about the JCAHO's ORYX program, call the JCAHO's dedicated ORYX telephone number (630-792-5085) or refer to the JCAHO's Web site (http://www.jcaho.org) for comprehensive information. You will not find "ORYX" on any of the initial pages of the Web site, however; the Joint Commission uses the generic term "performance measurement systems" instead. A particularly useful page is http://www.jcaho.org/perfmeas/pmgsi.html, which offers links to pages describing

- Attributes of conformance
- Communication guidelines
- Data quality principals
- Sample measure profiles for hospital, long-term care, and home care
- Sample measure profiles for behavioral healthcare
- Background for completing the hospital, long-term care, and home care profile
- Background for completing the behavioral healthcare profile
- ORYX data reporting requirements

Introducing the core performance measurement initiative

Although the initial goals of ORYX were met, the JCAHO experienced problems with the Core Performance Measurement process. Too many measures were initially approved (in the tens of thousands). The data collection system was unwieldy, statistics were questionable, and the JCAHO's approach to monitoring and intervention lacked clarity. There were also a fair share of complaints from the field about cost and labor to collect the data.

In addition, due to the problems encountered and the delay in initial implementation, the JCAHO created exceptions for smaller organizations and in the spring of 1999 capped the number of required measures at six and removed the "percent of population" requirement.

Hospitals must continue to participate in ORYX and should continue to seek low-cost and low-risk measurements that have meaningful relevance to quality and operations. You should continue to closely monitor the development of the core measures initiative and focus on early study and benchmarking of your clinical performance in the likely target categories.

The JCAHO has established the following initial clinical focus areas for hospitals:

- Acute myocardial infarction
- Community-acquired pneumonia
- Congestive heart failure
- Pregnancy and related conditions
- Surgical procedures and complications

The JCAHO chose these areas because they are high-risk, high-volume, problem-prone areas that relate to clinical performance, patient perception of care, and health status measures. Expert panels drawn from the hospital field assisted the Joint Commission in selecting these measures. The Joint Commission expects hospitals to collect data beginning January 2001.

Your response to the plan

What should quality directors be doing in response to the JCAHO's core measures plan? Consider implementing these ideas:

- Review the proposed measures to determine whether you already collect relevant data. If you do, consider how you might strengthen your performance in those areas and obtain comparative data to see how your hospital stacks up with others.

- If you don't collect data in some areas, begin to plan how you might do so at a reasonable cost. Even if the JCAHO eventually revises them further, you'll develop an understanding of the collection process and gain an understanding of your performance in key areas.

- Inform your senior quality committees of the new plan to help them understand its potential benefits and risks.

- Consider whether you would like to establish routine reporting for your quality oversight committee, and potential for the board, in some or all of the measures.

- Monitor developments and continue to prepare as this plan evolves.

Note that many of the measures use data not readily accessible from computerized data bases. If you do not have a robust clinical information system (and perhaps even if you do), it is quite likely that additional medical record review and data collection may be needed for some of these indicators. Become familiar with them now so that you can begin to assess potential resource implications if the indicators are adopted in their current form.

Pay attention to the specific data element definitions in the draft indicators. They may vary from your current approach to measurement, and you may be well advised to tweak your current PI program to measure using these definitions so that you begin to develop experience with them.

Part II

Managing the Performance Improvement Process

Chapter 4

Preparing for Survey: The Key Is an Organized, Ongoing, and Consistent Approach

Although the survey preparation process is arduous, complex, and sometimes frustrating, more than 5,200 hospitals and nearly 10,000 other healthcare providers have committed to follow Joint Commission on Accreditation of Healthcare Organizations (JCAHO) standards and strive to achieve JCAHO accreditation. Why? Because, although accreditation is not required by law, if these organizations wish to stay competitive, enhance their public image, gain managed care contracts, borrow money or float bond issues, and maintain Medicaid and Medicare funding, they must receive the JCAHO's "Good Housekeeping seal of approval."

Nevertheless, compliance with these standards benefits hospitals in more than purely financial terms. The standards require you to strive to provide high-quality care and, as a result, will help you better serve your staff, your patients, and your community. Quality care is not an option in today's healthcare market. Performance improvement (PI) is key to our patients, our community, and to the JCAHO. If you cannot prove to surveyors that you consistently work to improve all of your hospital's systems, then you will most likely not receive accreditation.

How do you ensure that your hospital remains compliant with the JCAHO's PI standards throughout the 3-year accreditation cycle? The key is an organized, ongoing, consistent approach to survey preparation. You need to

- Assess all PI documentation.
- Educate leaders and staff on the hospital's chosen PI approach and philosophy.
- Review the PI standards with key leaders and discuss the impact of these standards on leaders' areas of responsibility.
- Prioritize all PI needs to ensure that you focus on projects that will improve patient care and protect patient safety.
- Ensure that all measurements and assessments evaluate the level of efficacy, appropriateness, availability, timeliness, effectiveness, continuity, safety, efficiency, and respect and dignity of the process in question.
- Correlate all PI activities with JCAHO functions.

Chapter 4

Read through this chapter to learn how to ensure that your hospital meets all of these challenges and is ready for your surveyors' visit. It offers you descriptions of all the key survey sessions that focus on PI, and it teaches you what to expect in each session, who's involved, what documents are required, and how to meet surveyors' expectations.

Announcing their 2000 standards, the JCAHO also described their plans to revamp the survey process and agenda. A predictable survey agenda may become a thing of the past. The JCAHO will increase the information it provides to surveyors before they arrive on-site. This information will give the surveyors a more detailed history of the organization and its performance and will help to direct surveyors to hospital-specific issues. The surveyors will have more leeway in constructing or revising the agenda on-site. Be prepared for possible off-shift visits, random record selection, and an agenda tailored to the unique characteristics of your hospital. We will continue to see a focus on competence, credentialing, peer review, and patient rights.

This new approach further emphasizes the need for a continuous approach to quality improvement and JCAHO compliance. In addition, random unannounced surveys are now truly unannounced. The JCAHO has included aggregation and analysis (formerly referred to as assessment; standards PI.4 through PI.4.4) as key topics to be evaluated during random unannounced surveys. Usually, standards selected for a random unannounced survey—which occurs for approximately 5% of all hospitals at some point in their 3-year accreditation cycle—are those that generated the most Type I recommendations during the previous year. However, this standard traditionally hasn't been a source of many Type I recommendations. Including PI.4 as a topic for random unannounced surveys indicates the new emphasis that the JCAHO is placing on data collection and analysis, especially for sentinel events.

It also suggests that while surveyors may not have written many Type I recommendations in the past for PI.4, they might be dissatisfied with the level of data-driven assessment they currently observe. You might consider revisiting your hospital's assessment activities to ensure that your departments and PI teams are using sound techniques. (For more information on aggregating and analyzing data, see Chapter 11.)

Opening conference and performance improvement overview session

What to expect

These two sessions occur at the very start of the survey and are designed to familiarize surveyors with your organization. Key staff, such as your PI director, chief executive officer (CEO), executive vice president, chief operation officer, and director of nursing, should all expect to attend.

During the opening conference, you will be expected to briefly overview the organization and discuss its management structure, mission, and vision. This allows the survey team to gain a basic understanding of your hospital and the services it provides, and it sets the stage for the PI overview presentation. Many hospitals prepare quick slide presentations that highlight

- The organization's structure, mission, and PI philosophy
- The number of admissions, discharges, deliveries, and outpatient visits the hospital handles yearly

In addition, at the end of your presentation you should invite the surveyors to voice any questions they have about the hospital. This will help you set a congenial tone for the remainder of the survey.

FIGURE 4.1

Preparing for the performance improvement overview presentation

The PI overview presentation is one of the most important sessions on your survey agenda. Surveyors use this session to gain a frame of reference for their unit tours and interviews, and you want them to leave with a clear understanding of your PI process. The JCAHO places a great deal of emphasis on PI, and your leaders should be well on their way to meeting surveyors' expectations if they include all the following issues in their presentation:

1. A brief overview of your hospital's services, size, population served, mission, vision, and values.
2. The chronology of the history of PI in your organization, particularly since your last survey.
3. A description of your PI plan. For example, describe:
   - What you measure
   - How you conduct assessments and what tools you use
   - How you prioritize and implement improvements and what process you use, such as PDCA (plan, do, check, act), 10-step, or storyboards
   - How you gauge if something has been truly improved and how you monitor changes
   - How PI information flows through your hospital and how staff participate in PI activities
   - Who receives reports, what information you give to the governing body, and how it is distributed
   - Who is involved in PI in your organization
   - How you use customer satisfaction and risk management information in the improvement process
4. A few brief examples of PI at work, such as how you've incorporated the steps "plan, design, measure, assess, and improve."
5. A brief introduction of how you integrate, utilize, and communicate ORYX/core measures data.

Historically, the PI overview gave your hospital an opportunity to explain its PI approach to the surveyors. During 2000 and 2001, surveyors will begin to focus on the integration and utilization of ORYX performance measurement data during this interview. Specifically, the surveyors will have had an opportunity to review your ORYX data and they will expect to see how you have folded that data into your ongoing PI plan (Figure 4.1).

Previously, this session was scheduled to last approximately 1 hour, and it's still a very important introduction to your PI philosophy and methodology. However, as of January 1, 2000, the surveyors expect you to devote 30 minutes of this hour to discussion of your hospital's ORYX data. In other words, it is no longer just enough to comply with the paperwork requirements of the JCAHO's ORYX program. Now, the JCAHO wants to see how your hospital is actually using ORYX to improve its performance.

The PI overview was formerly one 30-minute presentation at the beginning of the survey. Now, the first 15 minutes is all your hospital will have to present an overview report, with the remaining 15 minutes allotted to PI achievements since the last survey. You can expect the survey team to focus on your handling of sentinel events and reduction of medical errors during these 30 minutes, and this may not leave much time for you to boast about your selection and achievement of quality goals. Be prepared with succinct and interesting summaries of accomplishments as well as a thoughtful response to the expected questions on

Chapter 4

sentinel events and medical errors. Finally, as noted, the remaining 30 minutes of the PI presentation will focus on ORYX.

To ensure that you thoroughly orient the surveyors to your PI philosophy, the scope of your PI program, and allow discussion time for the ORYX initiative, your presentation should (concisely) address how you

- Designed your PI model
- Plan and prioritize your PI initiatives
- Select which processes or outcomes you will monitor
- Measure and assess collected data
- Develop and implement PI action plans
- Monitor your improvements
- Educate and train staff and leaders on your PI approach
- Report your results to leaders
- Communicate key PI information to staff
- Ensure hospital-wide collaboration through the use of multidisciplinary teams
- Ensure that your plan meets the intent of the PI standards

You should thoroughly explain your hospital's structure and PI philosophy to the surveyors as best you can in the short amount of time allotted for this session. The amount of time spent on presenting versus reviewing ORYX data will depend on the surveyors, so be flexible. In addition to the information you provide them on your ORYX measurements, the surveyors will have a graphic display of your data submitted by your performance measurement vendor, as well as survey questions to be used.

Be especially prepared to respond to questions regarding some of the "hot" topics in PI (e.g., pain management, sentinel events and error reduction, restraints, and resuscitation outcomes). A complete and succinct response in this early session establishes a positive impression up front. Of course, you will need to substantiate your claims of PI progress during the remainder of the survey!

Remember that this is the first impression your surveyors will have of your hospital, and this is the information they'll take out into the hospital to validate. They'll look for evidence of a consistent, collaborative, and ongoing PI approach throughout your organization, which is precisely the reason why the PI overview session is so critical. You should ensure that when this session is completed, surveyors have a clear understanding of exactly how PI works in your hospital.

How to prepare

In the past, the opening conference and the PI overview presentation were not formal interview sessions, and surveyors did not ask you many questions. Now, holding your hospital's ORYX data, they will indeed ask questions, and you need to be ready with answers.

- How do you integrate the ORYX data into your current PI program?
- Can you give some examples of the groups that currently review, share, and analyze this data on a routine basis?

- Has the collection of specific measures allowed you to identify data trends and patterns related to patient outcomes?
- What processes have you put in place to address the problematic issues the data reveal?
- How will you assess improvement with these processes?
- How do these efforts at improvement fit with your overall PI strategy?
- How do you identify, investigate, and resolve sentinel events with improvement plans where appropriate? Can you give examples?
- What processes have you put in place to reduce medical errors? Are they working? How do you know?

During these sessions, the surveyors will still focus on gaining a clear understanding of your PI program and your hospital's mission. They will use the information learned in these sessions to develop their specific questions for leadership interviews, visits to patient care settings, the PI coordinating group interview, and the PI team presentation.

You should ensure that all participants are comfortable speaking about the hospital's overall management structure and PI approach. For example, the participants should be ready to respond to such questions as these:

- What quality model do you use?
- How have you been educated about PI?
- How are staff educated about PI?
- How do you encourage staff input and feedback on PI?
- How do you prioritize your PI initiatives?
- How do you encourage multidisciplinary cooperation?
- Do you consider PI to be an isolated activity designed to meet JCAHO standards, or is it an everyday management tool used within the hospital?
- Based on the hospital's strategic plan, what are the key processes in the hospital?
- Are you currently measuring, assessing, and improving performance in these processes?
- How do you recognize and report a sentinel event?
- Is your PI plan thorough? Simple? Flexible?
- Is the plan as relevant today as it was 2 years ago? Do you review and update it as needed?
- How do you utilize the ORYX data within your quality plan?
- Do you consider collection of the ORYX data to be beneficial or do you consider it to be an isolated activity designed to meet the JCAHO standards?

The best way to help all the senior managers and the CEO prepare for the opening conference and the PI overview presentation is to conduct two or three survey refresher sessions one to two months before your survey date. Many hospitals hold these sessions during senior management group or quality committee meetings and ask the leaders to practice making their presentations, answer sample questions, and discuss pertinent standards and the hospital's current level of compliance with PI standards.

You should also educate the leaders on the leadership (LD) and PI standards and ensure that they are familiar with the general intents and overviews of all the functional chapters in the *Comprehensive Accreditation Manual for Hospitals (CAMH)*. During these practice sessions, be prepared to help leaders formulate the "right" answers. Explain to them what the JCAHO is looking for in their responses, and help them understand how the standard applies to their area of responsibility so that they can tailor their answers accordingly. For example, if a surveyor asks, "How do you personally ensure that quality is measured, maintained, and continuously improved?" the director of nursing and vice president of medical affairs might respond by describing current process and cost improvements resulting from new clinical pathways, and the vice president of marketing and corporate planning might respond by describing key PI focuses that relate to assessing and meeting the community's needs.

Consider drafting a script for the PI overview presentation as well. Remember, this is the first impression you'll make on surveyors, and you need to ensure that all key points are covered (see Figure 4.1).

Do not leave this to chance. Use the practice sessions to discuss who should make the presentation, why certain elements must be covered, and what visuals should be used. Review the script during a timed final rehearsal a few days before the survey because the JCAHO expects this session to take only 30 minutes, and you don't want the surveyors to start off their day behind schedule.

It's also a good idea to provide the surveyors with a written overview of your PI program, which they can then reference throughout the survey. They'll use it to help them ensure that all PI documents, policies, and procedures are consistent with your PI philosophy and that staff and leaders are familiar with your hospital's PI approach as well. Your written overview should include

- Your organization chart
- Your PI plan
- An outline of your PI methodology, such as the PDCA (*p*lan, *d*o, *c*heck, *a*ct) or 10-step process methods
- Examples of key process improvements over the past 3 years, organized by JCAHO function to demonstrate compliance with standards while focusing on important patient care issues

Document review session
What to expect
The document review session is one of the most important sessions in the entire survey—and the one that requires the most extensive amount of advance preparation. Although the JCAHO now places more emphasis on interview sessions than ever before, it still looks to your documents to find evidence that your hospital complies with the standards. Surveyors use this session to orient themselves to your organization and gauge the hospital's compliance with a number of key standards. Generally, only the survey coordinator is required to participate in this session; he or she should be available to orient the surveyors to the documents and answer any of the surveyors' questions.

More important, this document library helps you to conduct a complete assessment of compliance. If you don't have a document or an example of compliance for every one of the standards, then you know where to start focusing your preparation efforts.

The surveyors will review close to 100 of your hospital's documents, policies, and procedures in a closed-door session. They'll take the information you provided during the PI overview presentation and verify that your documents support that philosophy. For example, they'll ensure that the following documents are present:

- Your PI plan, which will provide a description of your approach to PI

- Your patient satisfaction overview, which will describe how you meet the needs and expectations of patients and others

- Minutes from various PI or PI-related committees, which will highlight how you measure and assess collected data related to patient care and patient satisfaction as well as required measurements such as medication use, blood administration, or risk management

Figure 4.2 provides a list of all key PI-related documents.

How to prepare

Document preparation is a long and sometimes exhausting process, and you shouldn't wait until the week before survey to gather and organize your materials. Begin identifying, reviewing, and organizing documentation well in advance of the survey; ideally, you should familiarize yourself with and begin reviewing these documents approximately 1 year before your survey. You should ensure that all the required PI documents, such as your PI plan, are present, up-to-date, and compliant with all JCAHO standards. Personally review or have members of your preparation team review each and every document to ensure that it is pertinent; occasionally, people will turn in documents that do not relate to the standards or are out of date, and you need to make sure all documentation presented is relevant and current.

A detailed cross-reference of all your documents is essential to a successful survey. Surveyors have hundreds of pages to review in just 2 hours, and proper organization of your documents will help them sort through the material quickly. Organize your documents by standard number, chapter, function, and issue addressed, and include appropriate tabs and notations, such as the name of your document and its location, in your cross-reference and on your documents. All documents should be labeled exactly as they appear on the JCAHO document review list and in your detailed cross-reference. Be sure that each binder, folder, or other documentation holder is clearly labeled for easy identification. Some organizations choose to establish a color-coding system for their documentation, using one color for each function. Nevertheless, no matter how you organize your documents, your ultimate goal is to make this review as painless as possible for the surveyor.

Leadership interviews

What to expect

Leadership is key to a successful PI program and is therefore a main focus for surveyors. To empower your employees, you must lead by example. If your leaders embrace the hospital's PI philosophy and methodology, they'll set a good example for staff and prove that PI is a priority for your organization.

Chapter 4

FIGURE 4.2

Performance improvement documentation

Organize PI information for your surveyors in a binder. Be sure to include all of the following documentation:

- Table of contents.
- Summary or copy of the hospital's PI plan (PI.1).
- Description of your hospital's PI approach (PI.1).
- Description of your planning process for the development of a new process or service (PI.2).
- Required documents relating to the measurement and assessment of
    - Operative and other procedures (PI.3.2.1).
    - Medication use (PI.3.2.2).
    - Blood use (PI.3.2.3).
    - Patient needs and expectations (PI.3.2.5).
    - Appropriate quality control activities (PI.3.3.3). Although the JCAHO lists this as a measure to consider, quality control activities are required by several other regulatory agencies; therefore, it would be to your advantage to leave this as a required measure.

    The following documents reflect measures that are to be considered and not required. Remember that if your hospital decides not to measure and assess these, you should think carefully about documenting this consideration:
    - Utilization review (PI.3.2.4)
    - Staff's views on performance and improvement opportunities (PI.3.2.6)
    - Behavior management procedures (PI.3.2.7)
    - Autopsy results (PI.3.3.1)
    - Risk management activities (PI.3.3.2)
- Description of PI processes. If staff are involved in hospital-wide, cross-functional, and department-specific projects, describe (PI.1.1)
    - How projects are initiated
    - How the project leader and participants, including medical staff, are chosen
    - The approach used to complete a project and where it is documented
    - Who is responsible for evaluating the results
- Summary of major improvement projects involving staff (PI.1–PI.5.1).
- Work plan that tracks each project (PI.1–PI.5.1).
- Most recent annual review and evaluation of the hospital's PI program. Summarize problems and/or opportunities to improve those that were identified during the year. Include actions taken and evidence of their effectiveness (PI.1–PI.5.1).
- Copies of the following:
    - Monitoring reports used to identify improvement needs
    - Relevant material on assessed community needs and the target populations served by the department
    - External data or literature used to guide performance efforts
- Monthly review of patient care quality and appropriateness activities or services during the year, such as findings, conclusions, recommendations, evidence of improved care, and most important, actions taken to resolve problems (PI.1–PI.5.1).

Surveyors will review and assess the leadership standards in virtually every survey session—particularly the document review session, leadership interview, CEO/strategic planning and resource allocation interview, medical staff leadership interview, nursing leadership interview, and department directors' interview. They'll gauge how familiar your leaders are with your PI program and other PI requirements and will ask leaders questions such as these:

- How have you as a leader implemented your PI plan?
- Can you give some examples of the results achieved?
- Have these results had a positive impact on your patients, your community, your hospital?
- What is your definition of PI?
- How do you apply it to your areas of expertise?
- How have you worked with other leaders in the hospital to improve the organization's performance?
- How do you recognize and investigate sentinel events? What have you learned from them?
- How do you learn about medical error in your area, and how are you working to reduce medical errors? How do you know it's working?

During the leadership interview, your physician, nurse, and administrator surveyors will determine whether your hospital's structure and communication and management methods follow the JCAHO's standards of leadership, PI, management of information, management of human resources, continuum of care, management of the environment of care (EC), and patient rights and organizational ethics. Because this interview is scheduled at the beginning of the survey, the participants in this session (your CEO, senior managers, and other key leaders such as the executive vice president, chief of operations, chief financial officer, or director of nursing) should use this opportunity to further explain what was touched on in the opening conference and PI overview presentation. They should discuss how your hospital works to meets its mission, goals, and management and PI philosophies.

The remaining leadership sessions—the CEO/strategic planning and resource allocation interview, medical staff leadership interview, nursing leadership interview, and department directors' interviews—focus on evaluating the communication process among senior leaders and the nursing and medical staff's roles in PI within the organization. Again, the surveyors will assess collaboration among the hospital's leaders; they'll gauge whether your leaders work together to implement your PI plan and philosophy. The medical staff, nursing staff, and hospital leaders should be able to prove that

- They have a clear communication avenue
- They carry out the hospital's mission and values
- They assess the needs of the community and incorporate that information into all planning and improvement processes
- Their PI activities are interdisciplinary and cross the boundaries of your management structures

How to prepare

Unlike the PI overview presentation, leadership interviews are formal interviews, and participants should be prepared to answer surveyors' direct questions on the hospital's mission, vision, and strategic initiatives as well as its clinical, management, and PI philosophies (Figure 4.3).

To ensure that all of your leaders are prepared to field these questions, you should hold practice sessions beginning approximately 6 weeks before your scheduled survey. Prepare a

FIGURE 4.3

Sample questions and answers for leaders

The JCAHO requires hospitals to "do the right thing, and do it well." A hospital must have a concrete approach to continuous PI, and your leaders must be fully knowledgeable about your PI system. Use the following list of sample questions and answers to help prepare your leaders for survey and to ensure that they make a good impression on your surveyors.

Q: *How would you describe your hospital's approach to quality improvement/PI?*
A:
- Describe your PI plan and emphasize its link to the hospital's overall mission, vision, and goals.
- Discuss the methodology used by management and medical staff leaders to identify annual priorities for improvement.
- Explain how you make sure that important populations and processes are given attention in the PI process.
- Describe the governance model and how it fits the hospital's culture, stage of development, relationships, and priority needs.
- Discuss management responsibilities for PI.
- List the resources available for training, supporting data analysis, and data management.
- Explain how you integrate priorities and goals, offer support to committees and other PI structures, and benchmark your data.

Q: *How do you involve employees in quality improvement/PI?*
A:
- Every employee has the right and responsibility to identify opportunities for improvement through staff meetings and discussions with managers.
- Staff have opportunities to participate in teams or committees as assigned.
- Staff help collect data used to improve processes and systems.
- Staff are briefed on key quality indicators at least monthly.

Q: *How do you select processes to improve?*
A:
- Priorities for patients and other customers
- Institutional feasibility
- Customer satisfaction
- All high-risk, high-volume, problem-prone processes
- Highly variable and unpredictable processes
- Suggestions from benchmarks and literature

Q: *What are you doing to reduce medical errors? Have you read the institute of medicine report and the JCAHO's materials on sentinel events?*
A:
- Discuss your risk management program and your initiatives to ensure complete and timely reporting of errors and incidents.
- Perform a prompt root-cause analysis when indicated (preferably using the JCAHO's format).
- Identify systemic causes of error and design quality improvement solutions.
- Identify "near-miss" situations and use this information to design improvements.
  If at all possible, have a few examples ready to discuss. Remember that discussions with JCAHO surveyors may or may not be information protected from subpoena in your state. Discuss this with your hospital legal counsel before going into details on any individual patient care situation with a surveyor.

Q: *What processes and outcomes are you currently working to improve? Why did you select them? How are you approaching the improvement, and what is the progress to date? Where could I go to look at the data related to this improvement project? How have you learned to analyze this data?*
A:
- Review your departmental quality improvement plan for specific examples of improvements.

FIGURE 4.3 (cont'd)

- Focus your discussion on improvements made over the past year.
- Consider how specific quality indicators are monitored.
  Be prepared to describe in some detail how you look at data to determine whether a process is performing as you expect, or needs some further assessment or improvement. Discuss statistical and quantitative methods, benchmarking, or other approaches to the assessment phase.
- Identify which processes your department(s) are redesigning or improving.
- Consider improvements initiated due to patient surveys and/or internal customer surveys.
- Discuss how the PI team or committee has used information (e.g., graphs, tables, other analytic tools) to redesign an existing process, design a new process to improve performance, and meet patients' needs.

Q: *How have you educated yourself in the hospital's chosen PI approaches and methods?*
A:
- Personal education/programs/seminars/books
- Internal programs and workshops
- Employee newsletter articles

Q: *How is the scope of service defined, and how are important aspects of care chosen?*
A:
- Defined by customers
- Capabilities of the service (e.g., what outcomes or information will be provided to the patients based on the services provided)
- Community need (e.g., how the services offered meet the needs of the community)

Q: *How does the organization set expectations, develop plans, and manage processes to assess, improve, and maintain the quality of governance, management, and clinical and support activities?*
A:
- A strategic plan drives overall priorities according to hospital strengths and community need.
- The board monitors and directs priorities.
- The PI program is driven directly by customer needs or expectations.
- PI methodology ensures comprehensive analysis and pilot testing.
- PI committees ensure integration and appropriate priority setting.

Q: *How do you, as a manager, (1) integrate services of your department into primary functions of the organization, (2) coordinate and integrate inter- and intradepartmental functions, and (3) develop and implement policies and procedures to guide and support services?*
A:
- Integration may occur during the annual goal-setting process and through the PI priority-setting process.
- We coordinate and integrate departmental functions by paying close attention to customer satisfaction in patient care areas and support services. By working together through integrated goal setting, processes can be improved.
- The medical staff department chairman helps approve, develop, and implement policies and procedures.

Q: *How do you, as a manager, assess the qualifications and competence of personnel?*
A:
- Assessments are performed during recruitment, annual performance appraisals, union contract negotiations, and competency assessments.
- Many patient care areas have specific competency requirements and periodic competency and skills testing. The results of these and the annual performance appraisal process can help nursing leadership assess competency.
- The medical staff department chairman can use the information gathered on appointment and reappointment to assess competency of the medical staff.

FIGURE 4.3 (cont'd)

> **Q: How do you ensure that services are performed uniformly throughout the organization?**
> **A:**
> - Leadership establishes and helps implement policies and procedures that govern a basic standard of care and service. Leadership is also responsible for ensuring uniform basic competency of its staff.
> - Through performance appraisals, job descriptions, and competency assessments, we can define uniform performance expectations and apply them consistently through each patient care area.
> - This can be accomplished through the implementation of policies and procedures that govern a basic standard of care and standard of service.
>
> **Q: How do you foster communication among individuals and departments to coordinate and improve care and services?**
> **A:**
> - Regularly scheduled leadership meetings foster communication among and between departments. Other avenues for fostering communication include clinical path work groups and multidisciplinary planning and quality meetings.

summary presentation for your leaders on the leadership and PI standards and scoring guidelines, a similar briefing for medical staff leaders on the medical staff standards, and a briefing for the CEO on the governance standards. In your presentations, distribute interpretations of the standards for the groups and give them examples of how they are implemented in your hospital.

Provide the participants with a list of questions surveyors may ask and walk them through the entire set of questions (see Figure 4.3). Let more than one participant answer each question and encourage discussion and suggestions for additional answers or examples of compliance. Remember, participants should feel comfortable answering your questions even if they are not sure of the correct responses. You will learn as much from the group's silence or disagreement as from a correct answer.

Approximately 3 weeks before survey, schedule a second round of practice sessions. Go through the original list of questions, but this time offer them corresponding answers. Reinforce the "right" answers, and explain as supportively as possible why "wrong" answers are wrong. Add a few new questions to remind them that you cannot predict exactly what the surveyors will ask—you can only make a best guess.

Approximately 1 week before survey, hold your final leadership interview rehearsal. Ask the leaders questions, but do not offer any help with the answers. Let them use notes if they must, but insist that answers be put in their own words. Try directing questions at various participants—there's no way of knowing which person a surveyor will question. Surveyors expect all leaders to understand all of the standards, therefore, a board chairman may be asked a planning question and a medical director may be asked a financial question. Critique the session when you are done, pointing out any potentially problematic answers they gave.

Performance improvement team interview

What to expect

With your survey application, the JCAHO requires you to submit a list of six PI teams in your hospital and brief descriptions of the projects they've handled. It's from this list that the JCAHO will decide which teams will be interviewed during the PI team interview session. These teams should have worked on projects that were important to patient care, should be able to demonstrate successful results to the surveyors, and should be knowledgeable about the hospital's PI philosophy and its relationship to their projects. The JCAHO then evaluates the list of six and chooses three of those teams to make presentations to the surveyors on survey day. You should expect an increasing focus by JCAHO on teams working to improve outcomes and reduce medical error.

Your organizational liaison will let you know approximately 2 weeks before your survey which teams are required to participate. As you draft your list of PI teams, include teams that are in different stages of implementation on both clinical and nonclinical improvement projects. This will help you demonstrate the breadth and depth of your PI program. As you decide which teams to include on your list, consider the following points:

- Is the project consistent with our current services, our mission, our vision, and our strategic plan?
- Does the project have a direct impact on patient care?
- Does the PI team have data that can be displayed easily and effectively?
- Is the membership truly multidisciplinary (i.e., does it include staff from medical as well as other disciplines)?
- Did the PI team use any external comparative data?

Offer your surveyors only the hospital's best examples of compliance from which to choose.

Each surveyor will spend 1 hour with a PI team and discuss the team's performance and accomplishments. The surveyors will evaluate how each team

- Coordinates PI priorities
- Develops and implements PI initiatives
- Uses appropriate tools and techniques
- Monitors their results over time

Surveyors want to find out exactly how your PI process works and whether your teams are developing clear action plans and are making real improvements in your organization.

How to prepare

Be sure to educate your PI teams on what to expect from surveyors; if the team members don't understand what surveyors want, they can't make effective presentations, and your organization won't make a good impression. Explain that each team's presentation should offer surveyors definitive data to demonstrate that improvement occurred and include a number of charts, graphs, flow charts, and/or storyboards. The graphic displays should demonstrate that you collect and assess data and use it to make changes to existing processes or to design new processes.

Make sure they understand their role in the survey and help them identify their project's goals in a clear and concise manner. Hold one or two rehearsal sessions and lead them in a question-and-answer session to teach them the application of the standards to their jobs and the expectations of the surveyors. Remind them that with the increased focus on the interactive survey process, a good presentation is critical. Their charts and graphs should be attractive and clearly show how the process has improved. Similarly, the PI team members that present should be comfortable speaking—and that takes a few rehearsals for most staff.

Chapter 4

Performance improvement coordinating group interview

What to expect

Although the PI overview presentation offered surveyors a high-level explanation of your hospital's PI philosophy, and the PI team interviews focused on the nuts and bolts of specific PI projects, the PI coordinating group interview teaches surveyors exactly how your hospital coordinates all PI activities. They'll want to learn how you

- Prioritize measurement and improvement activities to ensure that patient care needs are met
- Gauge the effectiveness of these activities
- Allocate resources to measure, assess, and improve key hospital processes
- Involve the medical staff in all PI initiatives
- Report key PI information to the board
- Resolve problems when expected improvements do not occur
- Review PI activities for compliance with JCAHO requirements

The primary purpose of this interview is to ensure that the surveyors understand your PI process. You should demonstrate in particular your focus on meaningful assessment of relevant data, your integration of sentinel events into quality improvement (QI) as appropriate, and your understanding of the emerging focus on reducing medical error. The PI coordinating group should have discussed these topics on a regular basis, with concrete action taken and documented in the minutes to improve the hospital's awareness and improvement of these topics.

You'll need to set aside time to address surveyors' questions and any issues they may have identified during their visit to patient care settings. When this session is complete, the surveyors should be clear about your PI process, have no unanswered questions, and understand how your program complies with JCAHO standards.

Your hospital's PI director and those individuals responsible for coordinating and prioritizing PI activities (e.g., your PI coordinating group) should all be prepared to participate in this session. In most hospitals, management personnel from administration, nursing, the medical staff, and other key support services all belong to the PI coordinating group, but that is not always the case. The size and composition of your group ultimately depends on your hospital's needs and the services it provides. For example, at a small hospital, the PI coordinating group might include senior managers; the directors of quality, nursing, medical records, case management, and facilities management; and your safety officer.

How to prepare

The PI coordinating group will be expected to clarify any of the surveyors' misconceptions about your hospital's PI program or methodology during this session. Because PI is addressed in some form or other in virtually every survey session, and the surveyors may develop a number of questions about what they've seen, you should prepare your coordinating group in advance to respond to these issues. As the survey progresses, note any PI questions the surveyors develop or trouble spots they identify and update your coordinating group daily. They need to know which issues or gaps in compliance were identified so they will be prepared to address them.

To help prepare the PI coordinating group for this session, you should take the following steps:

- **Review the 11 functional chapters** of the *CAMH* with staff to ensure that they have a clear understanding of what the JCAHO wants.

- **Review the PI projects** already underway in the hospital and brainstorm about what quality issues the hospital should address in the coming year. Once the group develops a list of existing or proposed projects, match them to related functions in the *CAMH*.

- Inventory the hospital to **identify all PI projects** going on in each department.

- Review the projects, and **select the best examples** of compliance to present to surveyors. Make sure the projects you choose have data and are multidisciplinary and easy to explain.

- **Develop good visual materials,** such as storyboards and other charts, to impress surveyors and support your presentation.

- **Select excellent speakers** to present the projects. These individuals are your hospital's spokespeople, and they should be articulate, confident, and well informed about the projects' goals and strategies.

- **Hold practice interview sessions** to help the presenters practice, refine their material, and be constructively criticized by their peers.

- **Advise the presenters to be brief and confident** when speaking to surveyors. They should highlight the reason for the project, its design and data collection, the findings of data analysis, and the actions taken from that data.

Interviews with hospital staff

What to expect

PI will be discussed in visits to patient care areas, and any hospital staff member may be asked to answer surveyors' questions. For example, surveyors will visit approximately 50% of all patient care areas, including ambulatory and outpatient programs and clinics, anesthesia suites, emergency services, and pathology and clinical laboratories; and it is during these tours that employees may be asked questions related to their jobs and any job-related, environmental, and PI training they've received.

Through these staff interviews, surveyors ensure that all patient care is provided in a truly collaborative manner and is subject to PI. Staff can expect to field surveyors' questions in any of the following interview sessions:

- Patient care interview
- Patient and family education interview
- Continuum of care interview
- Medication use/nutrition care interview
- Anesthesia, operative, and other invasive procedures interview
- Ethics interview

For example, in the world of managed care and shortened stays, the hospital's approach to patient and family education is crucial to patients' well-being. Patients are discharged earlier and earlier, and they must know how to care for themselves and manage their conditions. When the surveyors question general staff, they'll be interested in learning more than just

Chapter 4

FIGURE 4.4

The mock survey

Because of shortages of personnel and high turnover of key management positions in hospitals today, staff and leaders are increasingly asked to take on new roles and responsibilities and may not have the time they need to study JCAHO requirements. Instead, it's up to you to gauge what compliance problems should be addressed in your organization by conducting a mock survey.

This is not a one-person job. To adequately assess your hospital's level of compliance with any of the JCAHO's standards, you should recruit a number of reliable individuals who clearly understand the JCAHO's requirements to participate in mock survey teams. These teams will function along the lines of PI teams and will be responsible for

- Reviewing the hospital's level of compliance with their assigned standards
- Collecting and evaluating all relevant critical documentation
- Implementing improvement plans
- Communicating compliance advice to staff
- Monitoring the results of their action plans

If documented appropriately, these activities can also be used to demonstrate to surveyors how you use multidisciplinary teams to improve your organization.

The teams should examine all areas of the hospital. For example, a PI mock survey team would be responsible for evaluating every department and service's compliance with the PI standards. They should gauge how well the hospital's processes meet JCAHO standards and determine which areas need improvements by considering the following:

- Which areas of the hospital need immediate action to address compliance problems?
- Which areas have excellent practices and policies? Which don't?
- Are there any hospital-wide practices and policies that should be improved?

Once the teams have synthesized and prioritized all of this data, they should develop corresponding improvement plans and target completion dates. Although many of the issues the teams will address will be hospital-wide compliance problems that need global attention, they may identify department-specific problems as well. For example, if the radiology department has deficient or incomplete personnel records, only that department can correct the problem. However, if the entire hospital appears to be unclear on your fire response plan, you should initiate hospital-wide education sessions to address this and other safety issues.

how patients are educated; they'll want to understand how the hospital has improved the way caregivers address patients' education needs.

How to prepare

Information. Education. Presentation. Practice. These four elements are key in preparing your staff for the JCAHO survey. You need to provide all staff members with a basic understanding of

- What a JCAHO survey is
- How it affects them
- What primary issues will be surveyed in their areas
- Questions related to the JCAHO functions they may be expected to answer
- Basic survey etiquette

Conduct mock surveys (Figures 4.4 and 4.5) to help determine whether your PI program is in compliance with all JCAHO standards. In addition, you should conduct practice interviews

FIGURE 4.5

Mock survey assessment checklist

Directions: Use this checklist to help you gauge whether your hospital is in compliance with the JCAHO PI standards. See Chapters 8–12 for detailed descriptions of each of these assessment items.

Plan (PI.1)
- ❏ Does the hospital have a planned, systematic, hospital-wide approach to PI? (PI.1)
- ❏ Are all PI activities collaborative and interdisciplinary? (PI.1.1)

Design (PI.2)
- ❏ Are all new processes designed well? (PI.2)

Measure (PI.3)
- ❏ Is PI data systematically collected? (PI.3)

Does the hospital collect data to identify improvement priorities, especially for important processes or outcomes (PI.3.1), such as
- ❏ Operative and other procedures? (PI.3.2.1)
- ❏ Medication use? (PI.3.2.2)
- ❏ Blood use? (PI.3.2.3)
- ❏ Patient needs and expectations? (PI.3.2.5)

Does the hospital consider the collection of data to identify improvement priorities, especially for those processes or outcomes that may be important to the hospital (PI.3.1), such as
- ❏ Utilization review? (PI.3.2.4)
- ❏ Staff views on performance and improvement opportunities? (PI.3.2.6)
- ❏ Behavior management procedures? (PI.3.2.7)
- ❏ Autopsy results? (PI.3.3.1)
- ❏ Risk management activities? (PI.3.3.2)

In addition, does the hospital collect data on quality control activities (PI.3.3.3) as they relate to
- ❏ Clinical laboratories?
- ❏ Diagnostic radiology?
- ❏ Dietetic services?
- ❏ Nuclear medicine?
- ❏ Radiation oncology?
- ❏ Equipment used in medical administration and the pharmacy?

Assess (PI.4)
- ❏ Does the hospital systematically assess data using appropriate quality control techniques? (PI.4.1)

Does your hospital compare the performance of its processes and outcomes over time? (PI.4.2)
- ❏ With up-to-date resources? (PI.4.3)
- ❏ To other hospitals? (PI.4.4)
- ❏ Against reference databases? (PI.4.4)

- ❏ Does the hospital intensively assess identified performance problems? (PI.4.5) Be sure to include attention to sentinel events and reducing medical errors in this section.
- ❏ Are all major discrepancies between preoperative and postoperative diagnoses assessed? (PI.4.5.1)

Does the hospital assess
- ❏ Adverse events occurring during anesthesia? (PI.4.5.2)
- ❏ Confirmed transfusion reactions? (PI.4.5.3)
- ❏ Significant adverse drug reactions? (PI.4.5.4)
- ❏ Behavior management procedures? (PI.4.6)
- ❏ The competence of licensed independent practitioners? (PI.4.7)

Improve (PI.5)
- ❏ Does the hospital systematically improve its performance? (PI.5)
- ❏ When individuals are unable or unwilling to improve identified performance problems, does the hospital modify their clinical privileges or job assignments? (PI.5.1)

(Figure 4.6) to teach staff how to answer surveyors' questions, discuss the care offered in their area, and speak comfortably about the standards related to their area of expertise. The primary benefit of these sessions is to alleviate staff's fear of the unknown. If they understand the process and are prepared to answer any questions surveyors may ask, your staff will feel far more at ease during the survey. The most common PI-related questions they may be asked include the following:

- What process have you improved within the last year?
- Why did it need improvement?
- What did you change?
- How is it working now?

Their responses will teach surveyors a great deal about your organization, including how well and how consistently they apply their knowledge of the basics of PI in practice.

Environment of care document review and interview sessions

What to expect

The EC standards mirror the PI standards in many ways: they require you to plan, design, measure, assess, and improve the environment in your hospital. Many hospitals even integrate into their PI plan their required EC plan(s) concerning

- General safety
- Security
- Handling and disposal of hazardous materials
- Emergency preparedness
- Life safety
- Medical equipment management
- Utility management

Compliance with these seven key issues will be assessed during document review sessions, building tours, and interviews with staff and leaders. Surveyors will want to see that you have worked to improve the environment in your hospital, and they will focus on such issues as these:

- **General safety** Do you have a safety program? Do you evaluate and change the program on a regular basis to meet the needs of your patients, visitors, and staff?
- **Security** Do you monitor security incidents in your hospital? Do you make adjustments based on these incidents to better protect your patients, visitors, and staff?
- **Handling and disposal of hazardous materials** Do you have a surveillance program in place to view actual handling and disposal of hazardous material? Do you provide education to employees at time of hire and annually to ensure their knowledge and safety?
- **Emergency preparedness** When was your last disaster drill? Did it go smoothly, and did you learn from it? What changes did you make to your emergency preparedness program to ensure the safety of your patients, visitors, and staff?
- **Life safety** Do you conduct regular fire drills in your hospital? How do you ensure the preparedness and safety of your patients, visitors, and staff?

FIGURE 4.6

Mock survey interviews

Everyone in your hospital, from senior managers to line staff, should be prepared to answer surveyors' questions, and it's up to you to ensure that each person is comfortable speaking about the JCAHO's requirements as they pertain to his or her job description. The best way to accomplish this feat is to hold mock survey interview sessions with individuals from each department of your hospital.

Your mock survey teams should conduct these interviews and focus on

- Evaluating how well everyone in the hospital grasps survey etiquette (i.e., how to interact with the surveyor)
- Teaching everyone what to expect from surveyors during the survey
- Gauging individual staff members' knowledge of the standards

Each member of the team should randomly select employees in each department and ask them general questions related to JCAHO standards such as these:

All employees:

- Describe your job and how it fits into the mission of the hospital.
- Describe how your department fits into the mission of the hospital.
- What orientation and education did you receive?
- Did it include information on safety (e.g., safety, security, management of hazardous materials and waste, emergency preparedness, medical equipment, utility management)?
- Are you involved in performance improvement?
- What performance improvement process does your hospital use?
- What improvements has your department made over the past year?
- Did any of these improvements involve multiple departments?
- How does your manager know that you are competent to perform your job?

Patient care staff:

- How do you address patient confidentiality, privacy, and security?
- What is your unit's role in multidisciplinary activities related to education, care, and treatment of patients?
- Describe your referral, transfer, and discharge process.
- How do you ensure that these activities meet patients' needs?
- Do you use patient input to determine performance improvement priorities?
- How have you developed standards of care, appropriate policies and procedures, and consistency in services across the hospital?

- **Medical equipment management** Have you had any equipment incidents over the past year? What steps did you follow to correct the identified issues? Did you make any changes to the overall program to ensure that this type of incident would not occur in the future?

- **Utility management** Are staff aware of all the utilities present in their area? Do they know how to use them and shut them off in the event of an internal disaster? What improvements have you made to the system to ensure the safety of the patients, visitors, and staff?

How to prepare

Because staff members may be questioned on the EC standards at any time, you should ensure that they have a basic understanding of all the EC standards, the hospital's safety program as it applies to their jobs, and how the hospital has worked to improve its performance in all of these areas. Many hospitals use "flash cards" to teach basic safety information to staff. These cards should focus on safety issues such as how to report fires, internal and external disasters, and security incidents.

Surveyors will also review your EC staff education processes and documentation. They'll want to understand how you educate staff about the seven elements of safety and measure their knowledge. This safety orientation and continuing education should be documented in personnel files or in departmental binders that include all employees in a particular department. You should also be able to demonstrate that you regularly test staff's knowledge of safety issues. For example, you might issue a written examination, hold oral examinations, or assess their compliance though direct observations (e.g., the use of a fire extinguisher).

To prepare staff for this session, hold a number of mock interviews and surveys (see Figures 4.4 and 4.6). These impromptu drills will help motivate staff and raise their level of enthusiasm for the survey preparation process. For example, surveyors might ask such questions as these:

- What should you do in the event of a fire in your area?

- Do you receive general safety education? Is this information updated regularly to address the needs of patients, visitors, and staff?

- Do you have a basic understanding of the hazardous materials program, the medical equipment management program, and utility program?

- Do you participate in fire drills, emergency preparedness drills, and disaster drills? How have each of these improved the environment for patients and staff?

- How have you planned for a care environment that supports all of the patient care services you offer?

Resource management interview

What to expect

Resources contribute to the success of an organization, and the JCAHO is very interested in learning how you improve all the various resources in your hospital, such as human, information, and financial resources. Without a competent staff, accurate information, and stable finances, a hospital cannot improve its performance and respond efficiently to the needs of patients, family, and staff.

Interview sessions such as the strategic planning and resource allocation, information management, medical record, human resources, competence assessment process, and medical staff credentials interviews will all focus on how well your organization plans, prioritizes, and improves its information resources. Senior managers in health information management, information systems, human resources, and the medical staff office can all expect to be key participants in these sessions.

The surveyors' main intent is to determine which human, information, and financial resources are key to your organization, and how you plan to

- Meet future resource needs
- Measure and assess
    - The performance of employees
    - The need for information in your hospital
    - The need for and allocation of financial resources
- Improve the utilization of these resources
- Offer employees ongoing education and training
- Measure staff's competence and report this information to the governing body
- Communicate important patient information manually or electronically
- Assess the needs of your internal and external information customers to ensure that you meet their needs

How to prepare

The best way to prepare for resource management interviews is to review the JCAHO's human resources and information management standards with the previously listed key participants in this session.

Make sure that documents that support your compliance with the standards are properly organized as well. Surveyors will want to see that you are following in practice what is written in your policies and procedures. Prepare for surveyors to ask to see documents such as your

- Information management plan
- Documents, minutes, and reports supporting the assessment of information needs
- Policies and procedures related to confidentiality of information
- Policies and procedures related to medical record safeguarding, content, and completion
- Documented process for managing human resources (definition of qualifications, job descriptions, and a system to evaluate competence)
- Staffing information
- Orientation and training information
- Policies and procedures related to staff conduct and rights
- Annual budget and most recent annual audit
- Strategic planning documents
- Documents, minutes, and reports that support the assessment of financial needs
- Policies and procedures related to the ethical use of funds and marketing

To prepare for these resource-related survey sessions, you should hold mock interviews with your senior health information management managers. They should be ready to answer such questions as these:

- How have you been trained in information management?
- How do you protect the confidentiality and integrity of information used in the hospital?

- How do you ensure that qualified and competent staff are providing care?
- How do you assess qualifications and competence of staff?
- How would you describe your organization's planning process and its relationship to your mission statement?
- How do you ensure that priority PI activities receive the appropriate financial resources?

Conclusion

It is important to remember that the key to preparing for the survey is to take an organized, ongoing, consistent approach to all your preparation efforts. This chapter highlighted some of the key survey sessions that focus on PI. This same type of approach can be used to ensure that your hospital complies with any other of the JCAHO's functions. Remember, achieving compliance with the JCAHO standards is just one benefit for your hospital; improving patient care and protecting patient and staff is the ultimate goal of an ongoing approach to compliance.

Chapter 5

Leadership's Role in Performance Improvement

As a leader in healthcare performance improvement (PI), what do you find most challenging? If you are like most executives today, you have a number of frustrations. You find the Joint Commission on Accreditation of Healthcare Organizations' (JCAHO) PI standards too vague, you wrestle with many competing priorities, and you have trouble focusing your hospital on PI projects that matter: obtaining multidisciplinary cooperation, and bringing improvement projects to fruitful completion.

You need to find a way to convince each department in your hospital to think of itself as part of the "big picture"—the total patient experience—and to persuade all hospital staff to work together to improve the hospital's quality of care. This is the basis for competent, effective PI and can be a difficult task, because it means overcoming distrust and long-standing barriers between departments as well as legitimate professional differences in focus. Each department and discipline has its own priorities, and they may or may not coincide. It's up to a hospital's leaders to encourage all departments to establish common priorities and to determine how staff can work together to make improvements.

But which hospital leaders are responsible for overseeing which improvements? Leaders are found at all levels of the organization, from the governing board to front line managers, and each of these individuals is responsible in some part for the success of your hospital's PI efforts. Together, leaders such as these are all responsible for the quality of the hospital's performance:

- The governing body
- Senior managers
- PI directors
- Medical staff leaders
- Line operations managers
- Quality champions

Each leader should encourage staff to take a multidisciplinary approach to PI and should offer them the knowledge, incentives, and training they'll need to effectively improve the organization. They should strive to help staff achieve both the hospital's broadest goals (e.g., "improve our services to the Hispanic community") and the hospital's highly targeted improvements (e.g., "reduce wait time in ultrasound to no more than 10 minutes").

Chapter 5

This chapter helps you to better understand what each leader's role is in PI, how he or she is expected to manage the PI process, and what challenges this individual faces. Your leaders must understand and embrace their critical roles in improving the hospital's performance, or your PI program cannot succeed.

Leadership performance improvement cycle

Both hospital leaders and staff affect PI. Leaders develop the framework or "big picture" for the hospital's PI system, and staff help implement these plans. These two groups must work together to ensure that a hospital's PI program is a success.

However, staff cannot begin making improvements to your hospital until its leaders have developed and implemented a directed, meaningful, and focused PI framework. Leadership's input and direction are critical to the success of the hospital's PI program, and it's important that all of these individuals understand exactly what is expected of them.

Previously scored in the PI chapter, the standards referring to leadership's role in PI (formerly PI.1 and PI.1.1) are now scored under LD.4.1 and LD.4.2. These standards require hospital leaders to participate in an active, collaborative, and interdisciplinary approach to PI. The wording of these standards has changed little, but their new placement indicates that the JCAHO expects leaders to demonstrate comprehension of, and a commitment to, your hospital's PI program.

The following brief synopsis of the leadership PI cycle is designed to familiarize you with leaders' general PI responsibilities. Once you've read through this section and are familiar with leaders' basic PI roles, go on to read about their individual PI responsibilities described later in the chapter.

Plan

All hospital leaders should work together to develop an annual, hospital-wide PI plan that meets pertinent JCAHO requirements. As these leaders set the hospital's PI priorities for the coming year, they should reflect on the hospital's strategic plan, last year's performance assessment, and various other data gathered during PI evaluations. Chapter 8 offers detailed information on this topic.

Design

Leaders must select a PI approach or model for their hospital. For example, they might decide to use the JCAHO's "Plan, Design, Measure, Assess, Improve" model, Deming's PDCA (*p*lan, *d*o, *c*heck, *a*ct) model, or Juran's model. Most hospitals select a PI model once and then refine it over the years. A discussion of how leaders should design their PI program and select their PI model can be found in Chapter 8.

During the design phase, leaders should also establish guidelines for training staff on PI and managing the PI process. Chapter 9 discusses the specifics of designing new projects. The hospital's PI plan must be supported by effective, motivated, and well-trained teams to be a success. These are ongoing responsibilities for leaders, and they should continuously look for new approaches to education, training, measurement, and evaluation. Refer to Chapters 6 and 7 for specific information on how to best train staff on PI and oversee PI teams in your hospital.

Deploying performance improvement throughout the hospital

Once the planning and design phases are completed, management, medical leadership, and hospital staff are ready to put the hospital's PI plans into action by forming PI teams. These teams are key to a successful PI program. Remember that all improvement occurs through effective work teams—not through management fiat; a wonderful PI plan does not, in itself, improve anything.

Each PI team will be assigned a particular problem to handle and will develop its own PI plan, conduct its own measurements, assess those measurements, and make improvements as needed. It is leadership's responsibility to oversee these teams and ensure that they make improvements. See Chapter 7 for tips on how best to manage departments and teams as they work to resolve problems in your organization.

Measure

In the hospital-wide PI plan, your leaders will have listed which key measures the hospital will use to assess this year's improvement priorities. Individual PI teams will conduct these measures, and it's up to the leaders to ensure that they are reliably and accurately collected. Refer to Chapter 10 for more detailed instructions on collecting measurements.

Assess

Data alone is insufficient to trigger change; the data should be assessed to determine what the hospital's true improvement priorities are. Staff should measure data on the hospital's improvement priorities listed in the PI plan and submit that information to hospital leaders for high-level review by the oversight quality committees and the governing board each quarter. See Chapter 11 for more information on this topic.

In addition to assessing collected data, hospital leaders should review the effectiveness of the hospital's PI program annually. This is mandated by the JCAHO and is discussed in more detail in Chapter 12.

Improve

Over the course of a year-long PI cycle, departments and teams will work to solve performance problems in the hospital.

In addition, as each year draws to a close, leaders must assess the effectiveness of the hospital's PI program and use their findings to improve it. This annual assessment is essential because your leaders must prove to the JCAHO that they have thought about the strengths and weaknesses of the overall PI process. For instance, surveyors might ask leaders to discuss changes in training, committee structures, or new information management tools introduced to help teams analyze data. See Chapter 12 for more information on how to manage this improvement stage.

Individual leaders' performance improvement responsibilities

Several types of leaders "make PI happen" in your hospital. The governing body and senior managers (typically the hospital's chief executive officer and vice presidents) provide high-level oversight and ensure that the leadership PI cycle (see previous section) functions effectively. This cycle is typically supported by a PI director, who may have a number of other areas of administrative responsibility as well.

Individual improvement efforts are led by managers, medical leaders, and other members of the hospital work force who, though not in management roles, serve as "quality champions" nonetheless.

All of these leaders have important and somewhat different functions and needs for support and development. The following information will help you to find out exactly what each leader's responsibilities are and how they can best be accomplished.

Governing body

Legally, by regulation, and under the JCAHO standards, the governing body is responsible for your hospital's quality of care. But, there are many different strategies the board can use to manage quality. In most hospitals, senior managers submit recommendations to the board on how to handle various PI issues. For example, these senior managers may propose answers to key PI-related questions such as these:

- Which senior executive should be responsible for overseeing PI in the hospital?
- How can medical staff and administrative leaders best work together to implement PI in the hospital?
- What PI responsibilities should be allocated to line managers? How should they be supported by the hospital's quality department?
- How much quality data should the full board review?

In addition, to meet JCAHO standards the governing body should ensure that

- Medical staff and hospital quality improvement efforts are integrated.
- Senior managers and medical staff leaders jointly approve the annual quality priorities of the organization—and that these priorities are derived from and linked to the hospital's strategic plan.
- All departments in the hospital consistently look for improvement opportunities by reviewing appropriate performance measurements.

Figure 5.1 provides a self-assessment checklist that governing board members can use to ensure that they comply with the JCAHO's standards.

The governing board must decide whether it has the time, expertise, and interest needed to review the hospital's quality monitoring reports as a full board. Frequently, the board develops a quality oversight committee to handle this role (Figures 5.2 and 5.3). This committee's chairperson should be a member of the board and should report regularly to the board on the committee's findings. Even though the full board will not be directly involved in monitoring quality in the organization, it will still meet JCAHO requirements if it regularly receives information on the status of key PI priorities and efforts. These reports and deliberations must, of course, be appropriately documented in board minutes.

Typically, the board decides which senior executive is responsible for implementing the PI program. This role is most commonly given to a dedicated vice president or an executive from patient care, nursing, or medical affairs, although in some hospitals a leader from risk management or information management may take on this task. All that matters is that a leader is explicitly identified as accountable for the overall PI program.

FIGURE 5.1

Governing board performance improvement compliance checklist

The governing board should regularly assess its compliance with these common PI requirements.

❏ Yes ❏ No   The board has approved the hospital's annual PI plan, including the organizational structure to support PI.

❏ Yes ❏ No   Meeting minutes indicate that the board has discussed the appropriateness of the hospital's annual PI priorities.

❏ Yes ❏ No   Board members have ensured that the hospital's PI goals meet community needs. (This can be as simple as a PI goal of lowering infection rates or enhancing patient satisfaction.)

❏ Yes ❏ No   The board monitors (usually at least quarterly) a focused set of measures for the major priorities in the PI plan and ensures that management and medical leadership monitors all JCAHO-required measures.

❏ Yes ❏ No   The board has discussed and approved an action plan for investigation, identification, and reduction of sentinel events, risk management events, and/or medical errors; the plan and its follow-up are documented.

❏ Yes ❏ No   Board members have read the hospital's annual assessment of the effectiveness of its PI program and can discuss how it has improved over time.

Senior managers

Senior managers, typically the chief executive officer and vice presidents, are responsible for painting the hospital's PI "big picture." They are explicitly accountable for what we have called the leadership PI cycle. For example, they must

- Establish key multidisciplinary, hospital-wide quality improvement goals each year.
- Ensure that a common PI model is used throughout the organization (see discussion of PI models in Chapter 8).
- Define the importance of quality and how it will be measured in the strategic plan and annual goals.
- Link the hospital's PI program to employee goal setting and annual employee performance reviews.
- Allocate sufficient resources in operating budgets to the PI program.
- Participate as assigned in the hospital's PI oversight committee(s).
- Review all key PI goals developed by their own departments.
- Ensure that all staff focus on broader patient and customer needs rather than on departmental issues.
- Encourage all departments to collaborate with each other as needed.

These responsibilities should be included in their own job descriptions and goals, or both, for each year. Figure 5.4 (p. 76) provides a self-assessment checklist that senior managers can use to ensure that they comply with JCAHO requirements.

FIGURE 5.2

Establishing a quality oversight committee

Often, the governing board does not have the time to manage and monitor the organization's PI efforts. In response, many organizations establish quality oversight committees to take on this role and report their findings regularly to the governing board.

This committee's responsibilities can vary from organization to organization, depending on a hospital's size and leadership structure. Generally, a quality oversight committee
- Oversees the development of and approves the annual PI plan and priorities
- Evaluates the status of PI priorities throughout the year
- Approves the annual PI program assessment
- Plans and oversees PI-related educational programs
- Reviews reports on the current status of quality measures conducted throughout the organization
- Intervenes if routine measurements or sentinel events indicate that the hospital has performance problems
- Convenes improvement teams across departments and disciplines to monitor their progress
- Supervises broader regulatory and accreditation compliance issues

The committee will need to monitor a fairly extensive amount of details and data, and the governing board should ensure that the individuals it selects to join this committee are up to the challenge. In many hospitals, quality oversight committees follow one of these models:

- A committee consisting solely of the medical executive committee. The major risk of using the medical executive committee as your quality oversight committee is that it may focus its attention primarily on clinical processes and outcomes and may neglect PI goals for issues such as improving patient satisfaction, administrative support services, or hospital finances. The hospital's quality director will need to watch this committee carefully to ensure that it addresses all relevant issues.

- Dual committees, one focusing on medical staff peer review and medical department PI, and one focusing on hospital administrative PI. Although this model is very efficient and ensures that committee members work on topics with which they are most comfortable, the split between medical and administrative issues may make it difficult for the committees to establish, monitor, and help interdisciplinary teams. Multidisciplinary teams may find themselves expected to report to both groups with unclear accountability, and this means that the teams won't know which groups or individuals are in a position to take action on their recommendations.

- A single committee consisting of both physicians and hospital administrators. This combined group should help to keep physicians focused on all hospital PI initiatives. However, it can be very difficult for a hospital to develop such a committee until it has proved to its physicians and leaders that they personally will not have to address JCAHO compliance issues in committee meetings.

None of these models are perfect. The key is to form a committee that is suitable to the existing interests, expectations, and capabilities of the hospital's leaders and its medical staff. And it should also be willing to improve the hospital's PI program over time.

Surveyors will expect leaders to be able to discuss both their hospital's PI model (see Figure 8.1 on p. 123) and key improvements made during the past year. Although these leaders don't have to know all the minute technical details of each PI effort in the hospital, they should be able to overview key initiatives of importance to the entire hospital, especially those outlined in the annual PI plan that affect their particular divisions in the hospital.

FIGURE 5.3

Model agenda for quality oversight committee

In most hospitals, either the board of directors or a designated PI oversight committee (see Figure 5.2) reviews the status of the hospital's major PI initiatives at least quarterly. Ideally, these meetings should focus on the following issues:

Status of Performance Improvement Priorities from the Annual Plan
Review all key PI teams and their progress, preferably via data reports with accompanying interpretations of the teams' findings and conclusions.

Suggested New Performance Improvement Priorities, Teams, and Projects
Review ideas for new PI projects. The hospital may require managers to formally present their proposals to the governing board or the PI oversight committee, or it may simply authorize managers to form their own improvement teams and report their progress to the board periodically.

Quality Director's Summary Report
Review a summary indicating that all JCAHO-required measures are being reviewed as necessary; this report may or may not include the actual data, findings, and conclusions for each measurement.

Other Reports and Recommendations
Depending on the committee's specific composition and charter, it may review reports on the status of infection control, safety, risk management, utilization review, peer review, and caregiver competence improvement efforts.

Special Presentations
Every few years, major committees, such as the medical records, pharmacy and therapeutics, infection control, and safety committees, may review their goals and accomplishments for the board. These presentations will not replace the routine PI data they must submit to the PI department.

For instance, the hospital's PI plan for the year may outline targeted improvements in patient satisfaction and turnaround time for reporting results. All departments of the hospital should have a clear understanding of their own roles in achieving these improvements; in some areas, the role will be indirect (e.g., in the information systems department, patient satisfaction might be affected by registration and billing procedures). A sensitivity to their colleagues' goals is essential. In the previous example, it would be important for the information systems department to treat the laboratory and radiology leaders as valued "customers" to support the goal of faster turnaround times.

Each leader's level of involvement in PI varies. One has overall responsibility; a few write, edit, or approve the hospital's PI plan; some may join or sponsor PI teams; and most review reports on key quality and performance measures in their area(s) of responsibility. But each senior manager should be involved in PI in some capacity, including those in nonclinical departments. For example, departments such as public relations, fund raising, human resources, or information systems may not have been required to focus specifically on PI in the past; today, however, they're expected to conduct performance measurements and develop improvement plans like any clinical department.

FIGURE 5.4

Senior managers' performance improvement compliance checklist

Senior managers should regularly assess their compliance with these common PI requirements:

☐ Yes ☐ No The executive can describe the hospital's primary PI priorities listed in this year's PI plan.

☐ Yes ☐ No The executive can discuss how these priorities are linked to community needs, strategic needs of the hospital, and national/regional performance standards.

☐ Yes ☐ No The executive can discuss his or her department's PI priorities and how they support hospital-wide goals.

☐ Yes ☐ No The executive can discuss in broad terms how various hospital resources, such as staff, training, and information management tools, are used to support the PI process.

☐ Yes ☐ No The executive can specifically describe improvements made by the hospital in the past year.

☐ Yes ☐ No The executive can discuss handling of sentinel events and medical errors at the hospital: systems for identification and investigation, linkage to quality improvement when root-cause analysis indicates this would be appropriate, and areas of current priority or opportunities for improvement.

☐ Yes ☐ No The executive can describe how he or she would like to improve the PI process in future, which issues he or she would make a priority, and why.

Performance improvement directors

Most hospitals' PI programs are supported by a quality department and led by a PI director. This department typically oversees PI in the organization and is specifically responsible for

- Helping senior managers identify the hospital's top PI priorities
- Writing and revising the annual PI plan based on those priorities
- Obtaining senior leaders' approval of the PI plan
- Maintaining the hospital's focus on its strategic PI priorities
- Monitoring the organization's compliance with all regulatory and accreditation requirements and conducting necessary self-assessments
- Overseeing (rather than implementing) all PI efforts
- Keeping all staff focused on their common goal—improving patient care
- Managing various technical services, such as
  - Abstracting, entering, and analyzing PI data
  - Coordinating and advising PI committees and teams
  - Benchmarking data and researching competitive/comparative practices and outcomes
  - Training individuals, teams, and managers on PI
  - Responding to managed care information requests
  - Interfacing with peer review organizations

FIGURE 5.5

Performance improvement director's performance improvement compliance checklist

PI directors should regularly assess their compliance with these common PI requirements.

- ☐ Yes ☐ No   The hospital's PI plan addresses the JCAHO's measurement, community needs, performance, and benchmarking requirements.

- ☐ Yes ☐ No   Well-prepared and effective departmental and team PI plans are deployed throughout the hospital.

- ☐ Yes ☐ No   The hospital's chosen PI model is appropriate to the hospital's needs.

- ☐ Yes ☐ No   Individual PI teams develop their improvement plans based on a thorough analysis of the performance problem.

- ☐ Yes ☐ No   The quality manager ensures that measurements taken for the board and various other management committees address the hospital's needs and JCAHO requirements.

- ☐ Yes ☐ No   PI teams have access to educational and technical support that will help them conduct reliable and meaningful measurements.

- ☐ Yes ☐ No   The quality manager ensures that leaders thoughtfully assess gathered data throughout the year, using statistical and benchmarking tools as appropriate, and review the hospital's overall performance annually.

- ☐ Yes ☐ No   The hospital compares its current performance to its past performance, PI goals, and community and national benchmarks as outlined in the JCAHO standards.

- ☐ Yes ☐ No   The hospital has an effective method of collecting information about sentinel events and medical errors, can demonstrate linkage between this information and quality improvement, and can demonstrate that its approaches are consistent with the emerging national focus on these issues.

- ☐ Yes ☐ No   PI training and consultation are available to leaders and PI teams to help them develop meaningful, effective, and resource-appropriate improvement plans.

- ☐ Yes ☐ No   The quality manager conducts periodic assessments of the hospital's compliance with the JCAHO's PI standards.

Refer to Chapter 6 for detailed information on the PI director's role in developing the hospital's PI program. Figure 5.5 provides a self-assessment checklist that directors can use to ensure that they comply with JCAHO requirements.

Quality departments must have appropriate hospital support, or they will not be able to achieve organizations' PI goals. For example, even in large hospitals, most quality departments do not have the time and staff to manage all of the organization's PI initiatives. They may oversee some of the hospital's key improvement priorities, but they will depend on individual departments to manage their own PI projects as well as other support functions. Common interdepartmental support may include

- The medical records department and utilization review staff to review the quality of patient charts and perhaps to abstract key quality indicators

- Management engineering to design and conduct work studies and statistical analyses
- Human resources to train employees in PI
- Marketing to conduct patient satisfaction surveys

Medical staff leaders

Medical staff leaders, such as clinical chairs and chiefs, and medical directors and officers, seldom have formal annual quality goals like other hospital leaders. Physicians are typically independent practitioners and not hospital employees, and they usually report directly to the governing board through the medical executive committee—not through hospital leaders. Therefore, they have historically considered their processes to be separate from the hospital's and not accountable to hospital managers. This has made it difficult for many hospitals to encourage medical staff to participate in hospital quality improvement teams.

Nevertheless, most medical staff leaders and individual physicians remain deeply committed to high-quality care for their patients, and many are willing to join quality improvement teams that will enhance these outcomes. If the hospital focuses on involving the medical staff in projects of obvious shared value, such as implementing clinical paths that reduce costs, improve outcomes, and meet managed care requirements, hospital leaders can expect the medical staff to increase their involvement in quality improvement initiatives.

The challenge medical leaders face, however, lies in convincing physicians to join PI teams that focus on nonclinical areas, such as improving patient service and satisfaction. For example, medical leaders should persuade physicians that issues typically delegated to nurses and hospital managers, such as reducing waiting times or improving communication with patients and their families, are also important. Physicians play a key role in all aspects of patient care, and improvement in these areas is virtually impossible without their collaboration.

Therefore, to truly support PI in the hospital and ensure that physicians actively participate in all PI efforts, medical staff leaders should

- Work with hospital leaders to select the organization's annual PI goals.
- Discuss these annual goals with the medical staff.
- Identify the medical staff's and the hospital's shared interests, such as an enhanced continuum of care, and discuss them with physicians.
- Encourage physicians to improve patient satisfaction with both clinical and nonclinical services, and remind physicians that both patients and other hospital staff members are their "customers."
- Participate in PI teams and quality committees and encourage other physicians to do the same.
- Integrate PI into the residency training program if there is one.
- Consider PI as a potential focus when developing research programs (e.g., research on physician communication styles that contribute to patient satisfaction, or research on staff training methods that contribute to reduced infection rates).

Figure 5.6 provides a self-assessment checklist that medical staff leaders can use to ensure that they comply with JCAHO requirements.

FIGURE 5.6

Medical staff leaders' performance improvement compliance checklist

Medical staff leaders should regularly assess their compliance with these common PI requirements:

❑ Yes ❑ No The medical executive committee approves the annual PI plan.

❑ Yes ❑ No Meeting minutes indicate that the medical executive committee discusses the appropriateness of the hospital's annual PI priorities.

❑ Yes ❑ No Medical staff leaders are familiar with the hospital's annual PI priorities and understand why they were selected.

❑ Yes ❑ No Medical staff leaders can describe the hospital's PI model and discuss how they have used it.

❑ Yes ❑ No Medical leaders can describe specific PIs they have helped to implement.

❑ Yes ❑ No Medical leaders can describe specific PI initiatives in which physicians have participated with other disciplines to improve a process and/or outcome.

❑ Yes ❑ No Medical leaders can explain reporting of sentinel events and medical errors to internal areas such as quality or risk management, can explain how quality improvement is used to reduce these risks, and can comment on the relationship of the hospital's program to the emerging national perspective on error.

Line operations managers

Quality is measured on the front lines of patient care and service; therefore, line managers, such as nurse managers, ultrasound managers, satellite pharmacy managers, or physical therapy managers, are integral to the hospital's PI efforts. Each manager is responsible for PI-related processes and outcomes within his or her own area and may be called on to participate in interdepartmental efforts to improve complex processes.

Although these managers may require leadership, training, coaching, and occasional policing from the hospital's quality department, they are still responsible for making quality a priority in the organization. Generally, they are expected to

- Identify their own departments' role in hospital-wide PI efforts.
- Develop annual plans for measuring and possibly improving important processes and outcomes within their own departments.
- Collaborate with other departments through PI teams, as necessary, to improve interdisciplinary processes or procedures.
- Educate staff on the department's PI goals and any relevant PI teams' progress.
- Fully integrate PI into everyday operations.

Figure 5.7 provides a self-assessment checklist that line managers can use to ensure that they comply with JCAHO requirements.

JCAHO standard LD.2 emphasizes line managers' responsibilities for maintaining quality. It requires line managers to develop plans and operating goals that emphasize PI. For example,

FIGURE 5.7

Line operations managers' performance improvement compliance checklist

Line operations managers should regularly assess their compliance with these common PI requirements:

❏ Yes ❏ No	The manager can describe the hospital's PI goals for the year and how his or her department can help achieve those goals.
❏ Yes ❏ No	The manager can describe how he or she has allocated resources, such as staff time and information support, to accomplish the hospital's PI goals.
❏ Yes ❏ No	The manager can describe specific improvements that have been made in his or her department.
❏ Yes ❏ No	The manager can describe collaborative improvement projects undertaken with other departments and/or disciplines.
❏ Yes ❏ No	The manager can describe specific measurements that he or she monitors regularly to ensure that processes and outcomes are "under control" in the department, with specific focus on statistical and benchmarking tools to assure meaningful assessment.
❏ Yes ❏ No	The manager can describe hospital initiatives to reduce medical errors (as appropriate to their department) and his/her role in these initiatives.
❏ Yes ❏ No	The manager can describe PI goals he or she would like to pursue and why they are meaningful to the patient or customer population served by his or her department.

they must consider such issues as these: "Is this the year we should expand our ambulatory service delivery? Is this the year we will introduce a new laparoscopic procedure? Do we need to reduce the costs of food and nutrition services?" Concrete annual goals such as these focuses attention on quality and performance in their areas.

Line managers must set goals for their employees, monitor their staff's performance, and coach them when needed. If these leaders use the hospital's quality plan and annual quality goals as a guide when developing their own departments' PI priorities, they will support the hospital's strategic plan and help the hospital achieve a seamless approach to quality. They should make this "quality focus" a requirement for every employee and evaluate it during annual performance appraisals.

Quality champions

Some of the greatest heroes in healthcare PI are individuals who do not hold management titles. These quality champions are found throughout our hospitals and medical groups. They are often skilled clinicians who take the time and energy to educate themselves about the processes of PI, who have a talent for data analysis, who possess strong communication and persuasive abilities, and who are leaders among their peers. They help lead PI initiatives in the hospital by

- Studying and learning PI methods
- Facilitating teams and managing group processes
- Serving as a personal model of continuous improvement and learning

It is important to offer these informal leaders sufficient orientation to the JCAHO standards and survey processes so that they can comfortably share what they know. Some organizations identify and support these individuals by providing basic quality training to 100% of their work force, including physicians. Others identify them through conventional management human resource processes, including monitoring physicians on medical staff committees, and offer them specialized training. The key responsibility of the hospital is to notice individuals with talents and interests in leading quality improvement and to make support resources available to them, including training, coaching, technical help, recognition, and allocation of time through careful goal setting.

Quality champions are likely to be interviewed by JCAHO surveyors in the context of the PI team interview. They are likely to be the staff who participate on the successful teams and who eagerly respond to inquiries about why a priority was selected, how the team knew that it had identified the root cause of the problem, what challenges were encountered in data collection and statistical analysis, how the group creatively developed improvement ideas, and so on. Knowledgeable quality champions, backed up by informed, involved leadership and committed staff, will secure for your hospital a dedication to quality that energizes every aspect of care.

Notes

Chapter 6

Implementing the Performance Improvement Plan: The Performance Improvement Director's Role

It's the performance improvement (PI) director's responsibility to oversee the entire improvement process, from developing a PI plan to overseeing all PI improvement projects. Once you've developed the hospital's PI plan in conjunction with the appropriate hospital leaders (see Chapter 8 for detailed information on how to develop a PI plan), you may feel "stuck"—not quite sure how to put your plans into action. This chapter offers you the practical advice and tips you'll need to ensure that your PI plans produce concrete results. It will teach you how to

- Prepare to implement your PI plan
- Create a sound infrastructure to support your PI efforts
- Oversee data collection
- Establish PI training programs
- Monitor the implementation of PI in the hospital

Where to focus and how fast to move

Before you can put your carefully made hospital-wide PI plan into action (see Chapter 8 for detailed information on developing a PI plan), you should

- Assess the hospital's critical priorities
- Assess medical staff and interdisciplinary relationships
- Assess management maturity
- Assess the hospital's current levels of performance
- Focus on both departmental and hospital-wide priorities

These factors will determine the speed and style of implementing your plans. By thoughtfully evaluating these factors, you'll be sure to develop a competent, successful PI program that won't become lost among too many overambitious projects.

Assess the hospital's critical priorities

In an era of ever more limited resources, hospitals must ensure that all chartered PI teams focus on issues that are true business imperatives—issues that affect the hospital's success or failure in a meaningful way. Lack of discipline at this point can lead to wasted resources and poor results.

Therefore, before you establish any PI teams, look over the list of hospital-wide improvement priorities in the PI plan and ensure that you have the resources to charter a PI team for each of these initiatives. You need to stay focused on the hospital's business imperatives and move smaller, less important projects to the "back burner."

Monitoring current trends

By keeping track of new Joint Commission on Accreditation of Healthcare Organizations (JCAHO) standards, as well as larger national discussions of topics such as medical error, pain management, and patients' rights, you can responsibly guide the hospital to the right priorities. This requires reading *Briefings on JCAHO* and tracking www.jcaho.org, www.aha.org, www.iahsc.com, www.nahq.org, and www.ncqa.org to become aware of hot topics early on. With this information you can begin to consider their impact on your hospital's priorities. Early awareness of hot topics and changes in JCAHO standards gives you more time to prepare to meet rising challenges.

For example, if you were surveyed in 1998 or 1999, by the time of your next survey you will face very different emphases by surveyors. Figure 6.1 details evolving issues in JCAHO accreditation. Prepare for these changes by continuously monitoring JCAHO and related publications and/or Web sites.

The Health Care Financing Administration (HCFA) is establishing new Conditions of Participation for Hospitals in Medicare: no facility can afford to ignore developments in this area, nor should they ignore major national research such as the Institute of Medicine's study on medical error. The political arena is also full of issues of importance to healthcare, notably the current discussion of a "patients' bill of rights." The American Hospital Association, your state hospital association, and other professional organizations, as well as the journals and Web sites previously listed can help you take an active role in your facility's response to such new challenges.

As the Joint Commission releases information about changes in accreditation standards, assess your current PI plan and your hospital's relevant processes. When you observe these changes moving closer to acceptance, either as standards, regulations, or laws, work with your PI committees to adjust the PI plan as needed to ensure that your priorities are in compliance. Your goal is to avoid a last-minute response when it may have been possible to build steadily toward collecting the right data, sharing with the right people, and making the right changes to respond to a new national or community need in PI.

Several issues took center stage in the late 1990s:

- Increasing responsibilities of leaders to understand how PI is integral to operations of a high quality hospital
- Treating pain as an integral part of patient assessment and treatment

FIGURE 6.1

Monitoring current trends

Review continuously the information described in this figure. Your PI plan needs attention to these challenges as you update it at least once a year:

Findings from Your Own Last JCAHO Survey

- Type I recommendations from last JCAHO visit
- Supplemental recommendations from last JCAHO visit

Findings from other regulatory visits, especially those that communicate to the JCAHO: state Department of Public Health, HCFA, etc.

JCAHO Standards Changed in Recent Years (Highlights)
1999

- Functional rehabilitation assessment, care, and treatment
- Patients' rights
- Use of restraint and seclusion
- PI—focus on design and redesign of new processes
- PI—required and considered measures
- PI—sustained improvement
- Sentinel events—monitoring, reporting, improved performance, and risk reduction

2000

- Pain management
- Resuscitation
- Leadership standards for clinical practice guidelines
- PI—required and considered measures
- Patients' rights
- Restraint and seclusion
- Medication use
- ORYX data focus

Potential Changes for 2001

- Revision of medical staff chapter
- Revision of standards related to anesthesia
- Increased ORYX focus, core performance measures
- Public disclosure issues

National Topics

- Institute of Medicine study on medical errors
- Related legislative, research, and association proposals for improvement
- Patient rights
- Pain management

Other Regulatory Issues

- State regulations—existing, new, and proposed
- Federal regulations—existing, new, and proposed (especially HCFA conditions of participation)

Chapter 6

- Minimizing the use of restraints and using them only within a process tightly controlled by new mandates from the HCFA and the JCAHO
- A new relationship between patient and hospital, with greater emphasis on patient participation and even leadership in the clinical decision-making process
- The high incidence of medical errors, even in the absence of high-profile sentinel events
- The need for managers at all levels to understand competent data assessment and basic statistical tools, so that PI activities are well-targeted and effective

The PI director will face these new challenges aware of the continuing JCAHO focus on "the basics"—we cannot allow our measurement, education, and improvement efforts to wither in the fundamentally important areas of staff competence, safety, infection control, patient care practices, etc.

Assess medical staff and interdisciplinary relationships

Even the most collegial relationships among the medical staff and other disciplines can be strained when PI teams begin to challenge the status quo and question long-standing practices and prerogatives. It is important to recruit experienced and mature facilitators to help work through these issues. In addition, the facilitator and hospital leaders should be prepared to spend whatever time is necessary with medical leadership at every step of the process to ensure that there is solid consensus and understanding as the process improvement takes shape.

Also, it's always a good idea to tackle only one highly politicized process at a time so that the medical staff doesn't feel overwhelmed or under attack. Or if medical staff relationships are very poor in a given area, a PI team may not be feasible or desirable at all. For instance, if a group of surgeons and anesthesiologists are at war over scheduling priorities, it would be wise to work out those issues before you assign a PI team to develop a comprehensive process improvement on operating room utilization and turnover.

Assess management maturity

You should take the time to gauge whether the hospital's department managers are experienced enough in PI to help lead PI initiatives and oversee data measurement, collection, and assessment. Highly experienced and seasoned managers may be able to conduct routine monitoring and evaluation activities without difficulty. Those who know their processes and services well and have been engaged in measurement before will be able to define their programs' priorities, select key measures, and implement measurement through routine operations. For example, a radiology manager may quickly settle on wait times, report turnaround times, and film reread error rates as critical issues, and he or she may be able to integrate daily record keeping in such a way that these data are produced routinely with little additional effort.

Managers who are newer to their programs or level of responsibility may find measurement technically overwhelming and professionally threatening until they are more comfortable with their scope of operational responsibility. Therefore, it is important for you to design a PI program that supports and nourishes both experienced and inexperienced managers. This program should encourage all managers to develop their skills and contribute effectively over time to the hospital's improvement efforts. The program may include technical support resources and training as well as a systematic orientation for the newer managers that perhaps includes a monthly review and coaching session.

By the same token, as you select managers and staff to join PI teams, you should be sensitive to each individual's varied background and maturity level. Training and workshops for PI teams should address these different skill levels and work to identify each individual's strengths.

Assess the hospital's current levels of performance

Be sure to assess the hospital's current level of performance to determine which areas are in the greatest need of improvement before you charter any PI teams. For example, if current measures indicate that the hospital has a serious quality problem in a certain area, you should focus the hospital's attention on that issue. Processes with a higher level of operational quality can be moved to the side until the hospital's major problems have been conquered.

Ideally (and as envisioned under the JCAHO standards), the hospital's annual self-evaluations and goal setting will incorporate all available data, including risk and claims data, patient satisfaction information, clinical and technical outcomes, competitive and comparative benchmarks wherever available, and market research. These data will help you to determine which areas are performing well and which areas must be improved.

Focus on departmental and hospital-wide priorities

Every hospital should focus its improvement efforts on both departmental and hospital-wide improvement priorities. But although it's important to focus on some departmental issues, a sophisticated organization seeks to limit its investment in departmental PI efforts to ones that meaningfully reflect performance and can genuinely trigger corrective action. In addition, you should also be extremely selective about the number and type of teams you charter to work on complex processes, preferring a few groups invested in improvement of processes of compelling importance to patient care or other critical priorities.

Whether an improvement effort is focused on a single department or on many disciplines, you should ensure that each improvement priority will truly help improve patient care, service, support processes, and won't be a needless drain on the hospital's resources.

Creating a sound performance improvement infrastructure

As discussed in Chapter 5, the hospital's leaders are responsible for developing the groundwork for the PI program. Each year, they meet to

- Establish the hospital-wide PI plan
- Select a PI approach or model
- Establish PI support structures, such as committees, training sessions, and information management support
- Select a number of key measures the hospital must take to meet JCAHO requirements and advance the hospital's own improvement priorities
- Assess the data gathered by PI teams for these key measures
- Develop improvement plans for key hospital improvement priorities that matter to patients and other customers

However, the hospital's leaders cannot accomplish all of these tasks on their own; they'll need PI teams to implement their plans and manage day-to-day activities. For example, these teams will collect data, make initial assessments of the gathered data, develop creative improvement plans for leadership's review, and pilot test and implement the approved plans. Some of these initiatives will occur within individual departments, and others will involve multiple departments and disciplines.

As the hospital's PI director, you should ensure that the hospital solidly supports PI so that both department and team initiatives are successful. It's your responsibility to ensure that leadership's "big picture" is a top priority for the entire hospital and that each staff member understands exactly what his or her role is in the improvement process. These individuals should know concretely what their departments can do and what their PI goals specifically will be.

In addition, you must help each department manager to establish formal targets and goals. Although there is no JCAHO requirement specifically indicating that managers should be reviewed on the basis of their fulfillment of their PI plans, standard LD.2 does speak to the responsibility of managers to lead and participate in PI initiatives. Typically, each manager should establish performance goals, including quality targets, that will form the foundation for their annual reviews and, possibly, incentive or merit increases. Like other departmental goals, these may be fulfilled by the manager alone, through the efforts of teams within the department, and/or by teams whose members are drawn from multiple departments and disciplines.

Conducting departmental self-evaluations

You must ensure that each and every department in the hospital assesses its key processes and identifies which of them are "high volume, high risk, and problem prone." In addition, each department must understand how to conduct measurements that are consistent, appropriate, and compliant with JCAHO requirements.

This is not an easy task. Each department will need a great deal of guidance and coaching from you, and you'll need to ensure that each department's program is well integrated with all of the hospital's other priorities and skills. The best way to handle this dilemma is to establish a simple, clear, annual process that requires each department to describe itself and its core processes (thereby also meeting leadership standards requiring a "scope of service" for each department) each year, and to establish some basic measurements that should be conducted for various important processes, per JCAHO requirements. Figure 6.2 provides a list of recommended steps you can follow to accomplish this.

Forms and information flow

To effectively coordinate the PI program, you will want to use a consistent format for all departments' PI planning efforts. See Figures 6.3, 6.4, and 6.5 for sample forms you can use to collect basic information on each department's leadership structure, scope of services, and planned measures. These sample forms have been designed to fit together well, to be easy to use, and to contain just what is needed; there is nothing extraneous. In your hospital, you might need to add other components to make the forms work within your structure, but you can use these as a starting point.

FIGURE 6.2

Conducting a departmental performance improvement self-assessment

This brief overview summarizes the steps involved in developing an effective and standards-compliant departmental PI plan. Figures 6.3 and 6.4 contain sample forms that can make the process more consistent and complete.

Step 1: Ask each department to prepare an annual description of who they are, whom they serve, and what they do.
In this description, each hospital and medical staff department should describe its leadership structure and scope of services (required under LD.2) and classify which part of the care and service it offers are high risk, high volume, or problem prone (PI.3.4).

Step 2: Ask each department to establish how it will measure its important processes.
Each department should select specific measures it will use to ensure that core services and processes operate within desired parameters. When applicable, patient (or other customer) satisfaction should be one of these measures.

Step 3: Ask each department to decide which members will participate in improvement teams.
Each department may participate in one or more PI teams, on either departmental projects or multidisciplinary issues chartered by the PI oversight committee. It will be these teams that conduct measures to monitor the process being evaluated, changed, or improved. Chapter 7 contains more information on working effectively with teams.

Implementing the program

As discussed in Chapter 5, it is imperative that PI be fully integrated into the routine of every manager, including medical leaders. What you want to avoid is the "Friday is quality day" syndrome or "we deal with quality at our committee" response. Continuous performance management and improvement should be every leader's goal, and the PI program should provide the tools to support them.

How can you make this happen? Here are some specific tips on implementation:

1. Ensure that PI is explicitly referenced in all management job descriptions in the hospital or that there is a clearly communicated statement to all managers that PI is implicit in every job. Another way to do this is to include involvement in PI as a criterion for evaluating the performance of managers during formal annual performance reviews.

2. Ensure that the PI oversight committee and senior managers endorse the principle that every manager will conduct an annual PI planning exercise. Each year, have the PI oversight committee formally approve a timetable for PI plans to be developed and submitted by each department.

3. Hold brief orientation sessions for all managers, and continue to offer these sessions as new managers join the hospital. These sessions should discuss how to plan for PI and how the PI process will help them achieve their goals of delivering measurable

FIGURE 6.3

Identifying a department's performance improvement priorities

Directions: Use this form to help you determine what each department's PI priorities are.

Department name:

_____

_____

Describe how the department's strategic goals and mission further the hospital's strategic goals and mission.

_____

_____

List the department's internal customers (e.g., physicians, hospital staff) and external customers (e.g., patients, families, payers).

_____

_____

Describe the department's scope of care/services. What processes, procedures, and services are performed? Which types of practitioners or workers provide these services? At what sites and at what times are these services provided?

_____

_____

Which of these services are high volume, high risk, problem prone, high profile, or cross functional?

_____

_____

How do these processes perform compared to professional standards and benchmarks?

_____

_____

How do you plan to monitor your most important processes for quality? What measures will you take?

_____

_____

FIGURE 6.4

Planning for measurement

Directions: Use this form to help you plan out each department's performance measures. You should note which measures will be taken, what your performance goals are for each, specifically how each process will be measured, and which JCAHO functions and dimensions of performance with which each measure complies. Chapter 10 contains a detailed discussion of the JCAHO's requirements for mapping your measures to its functions and dimensions of performance.

Name of measure	How it will be measured	Frequency of measurement	Performance goals	Applicable JCAHO function(s)	Applicable JCAHO dimensions of performance

FIGURE 6.5

Measurement data report

Directions: Use this form to help you synthesize the data you collect on each measure and determine whether the process in question is performing well or should be improved.

Name of process, measure, or indicator:
_____
_____

History of the process (i.e., why is this process important?):
_____
_____

Goals for the measure:
_____
_____

Description of current levels of performance:
_____
_____

Description of trended levels of performance over time:
_____
_____

Findings and conclusions:
_____
_____

Improvement strategies/recommendations (list both what the recommended action is and when it should be implemented):
_____
_____

Plans for follow-up/monitoring:
_____
_____

FIGURE 6.6

Orientation to performance improvement planning for managers and medical leaders

An orientation to the hospital's PI program is typically provided by the PI director to all new managers and medical staff leaders. The following is a suggested outline for such an orientation.

Outline
- Why we do PI: our mission and definition of quality and performance
- JCAHO and other regulatory issues in PI that affect us
- How we define "who we are," "whom we serve," and "what we do"
- How we select what we will measure
  - High-risk, high-volume, problem-prone processes
  - Processes that are important for furthering the hospital's strategic priorities
  - Processes that must be measured to meet JCAHO and other regulatory requirements
- How we conduct measurement
  - How the quality department can help design and carry out measurement
- How we conduct assessment
  - How the quality department can assist with statistical and analytic resources
  - How to choose benchmarks and comparison groups
  - How to compare our performance to the literature, to that of our peers, and to our past performance
- How we perform improvement activities
  - How to set up a PI team and when that is appropriate
  - Our model for PI process improvements (e.g., PDCA, PDMAI, etc.)
  - Technical support available for team facilitation, data and information management, etc.
  - How we develop recommendations to improve processes and who can approve them
  - How we assess our improvement efforts over time
- Your responsibilities as a manager
  - Development of an annual PI plan that fits with the hospital's top priority goals for the year
  - Ongoing measurement and assessment
  - Communication with staff
  - Determination when improvement is necessary, and leadership of the process
  - Reporting to the PI oversight committee and others as appropriate
  - Annual self-assessment of your PI efforts
- Summary of how the quality department is here to help you
- Questions and answers

high-quality care and service. See Figure 6.6 for a sample agenda for such a session. A sample manager training handbook is discussed in Figure 6.7.

4. Encourage managers to stay focused on high-risk, high-volume, and problem-prone areas rather than diffusing their energies among too many quality measures. This is best done in two phases: first, by carefully orienting managers to the hospital's PI process before they develop their plans; and second, by reviewing the plans as they are completed and submitted and making recommendations for streamlining or improvement.

5. Try to help managers to move beyond traditional thinking about "quality assurance" that focuses on counting problems or defects (e.g., "We only do this for JCAHO," "Just pick measures you'll look good on," "Pick things that are easy to measure").

FIGURE 6.7

Outline of a performance improvement training handbook for managers

The following is an outline of the PI training handbook our hospital created to support new managers and teach them how best to implement PI in their departments. Although this handbook will become a valuable resource for your hospital's managers, you should remember that it is not a substitute for quality department resources, coaching, or counseling.

Table of Contents
Introduction: Letter to managers

Chapter 1:   Performance improvement as a management tool

Chapter 2:   Review of the hospital's basic performance improvement philosophy and structure

- The hospital's mission, leaders, and customers
- The strategic plan drives quality definitions and priorities
- Management goals for quality
- Quality monitoring and process improvement
- Performance improvement definitions
- Training for quality monitoring and improvement
- Is this "monitoring" or "process improvement"?
- Integration of performance improvement with the performance management process
- Integration of performance improvement with budgeting and resource allocation.

Chapter 3:   Quality reporting and communications

- The importance of communications in performance improvement
- Orientation of new employees to quality
- Conducting and documenting meetings
- Quality meeting agendas
- Model agenda
- Model materials for meeting preparation
- Holding the quality meeting
- Efficient, comprehensive, and effective documentation
- Minutes for a quality meeting
- Model documentation of a meeting
- Sample department quality meeting agenda, materials, and minutes
- Record keeping

Chapter 4:   Baseline monitoring and routine analysis

- Measurement basics
- Basics of data analysis
- When a baseline monitor might lead to a process improvement effort
- Common pitfalls

Chapter 5:   Process improvement basics

- Is this process a performance improvement issue at all?
- Selecting a process for improvement
- Why is a stable process better than a variable one?
- Developing a process improvement opportunity statement and plan
- Establishing a viable process improvement team
- Common pitfalls
- Tactical and operational problem-solving model

FIGURE 6.7 (cont'd)

Appendix A: Data analysis and statistical tools

- Overview of common data analysis tools
- Run charts
- Control charts
- Brainstorming
- Cause-and-effect diagrams
- Data collection tool design and check sheets
- Pareto diagram
- Costs of poor quality and benefit-cost analysis
- Flow charts
- T-tests and analysis of variance
- Action planning

Appendix B: Educational and support resources for performance improvement

---

This is best done in the orientation session and through continuous discussion and dialogue with managers over time as they improve their PI programs.

6. Introduce educational opportunities that will help managers think about processes that matter to patients and other customers and that will help them lead improvement teams productively and efficiently.

7. Set a deadline for annual planning to be completed (which should be approved by the PI oversight committee, as noted previously), and set and monitor reporting time frames to create and maintain the discipline of regular data analysis and interpretation. Most often, departments perform routine performance measurement and communication with staff monthly and may provide updates or reports on progress to the quality department and PI oversight committee quarterly.

8. Set deadlines and provide guidance and coaching for the annual self-assessment process (see Chapter 12 for more on this topic).

Overseeing your performance improvement program's data collection

Although it is not within the scope of this book to detail all of the nuts and bolts associated with running a PI program, the following tips will help you design the technology for your program in a way that is more likely to support JCAHO compliance.

To make real improvements, you need to be able to take reliable and meaningful measurements and make some sense of them. Therefore, you should ensure that your hospital has some core resources to help departments and teams

- Design data collection
- Develop reliable data collection methods
- Evaluate collected data to identify trends and significant changes

Chapter 6

FIGURE 6.8

What the hospital's performance improvement director should know about data collection and evaluation

The PI director should understand clearly all of the issues associated with data collection and evaluation to advise managers and medical leaders on the development and implementation of a competent PI program. For example, this individual should be familiar with the following issues:

Data Collection
- What measures are required by the JCAHO (Chapter 10 offers detailed information)
- How to design and use data collection tools, such as
  - Check sheets for retrospective evaluation of patient medical records and other documents
  - Log sheets for process measurement
  - Clinical pathways and variance reporting tools
- How to train staff to collect data
- How to identify and correct biases in the data
- How to evaluate inter-rater reliability and consistency
- How to handle situations of apparent bias or sabotage in the data (both through your human resources process and through the statistical process—e.g., when to discard suspect data from the data set)

Data Evaluation
- How to work with descriptive statistics (e.g., means, standard deviations, coefficients of variation)
- How to use statistical process control (e.g., construction of run charts and confidence intervals)
- How to develop charts and graphs (e.g., Pareto charts, histograms and bar charts, scatterplots, pie charts, trend lines, and, possibly, regression lines)

Figure 6.8 provides an overview of the basic knowledge and skills in data management needed by the PI director.

Designing data collection

Data collection is a very important and difficult part of the PI process. For example, at least one of the following scenarios is probably familiar to your hospital.

- A department wants to measure waiting time. It implements a sign-in log for patients and compares each patient's arrival time to the actual time the patient is seen. When the department starts to review the data, the staff members realize that they never articulated their goal clearly: Do they want to promise to see every patient within 10 minutes of arrival or within 10 minutes of scheduled appointment time? They did not collect the data correctly if they wanted to measure the latter.

Conclusion: *The department needs objective help in designing data collection tools to ensure that it has a clearly articulated measurement goal before it takes the time and energy to collect data.*

- Another department wants to measure the reasons for service delays. A log sheet is designed to capture steps that were or were not correctly executed to serve the patient on time. Department members begin to snipe at each other and divide into factions that are eager to find "defects" in each other's portion of the process, believing that they will thus be relieved of any personal responsibility for any overall process problems.

Conclusion: *Measurement itself should be as objective as possible and implemented in a team climate so that it does not simply become another vehicle for staff sabotage. If possible, data should be collected in a neutral method (e.g., a computer system that produces data as a by-product of routine patient registration, treatment, or record-keeping functions.) Resources must be available within the hospital to coach managers through these difficult stages of team development.*

- Caregivers recognize that it is important to meet patients' need for education and information about their care. They decide to measure their success in providing this information by reviewing charts to ensure that they correctly documented that they provided the patients with information and that the patients verbalized understanding. They are perplexed when patient satisfaction scores on information about care continue to decline.

Conclusion: *We need to measure the "dimensions of performance" that matter to the patient or other customer rather than conduct measures that are convenient or comfortable to us as professionals. Documentation is a favorite measurement source for hospital staff, and it certainly has its place; but the patient's technical and perceptual outcome is the real goal, and some measures must be in place to evaluate it directly.*

- We want to compare waiting time at our hospital to that at a sister hospital in a particular department. When we study the data we've collected, we are pleased to see that our waiting times are consistently shorter—so we can't understand why the other hospital's patient satisfaction is high with waiting time in their department while ours is low. On further analysis, it turns out that we are measuring waiting time to usher the patient to an examination room, but the other hospital is measuring waiting time to see a doctor. In our hospital, our problem is that patients wait a long time in the examination room before they see a physician.

Conclusion: *We need to ensure that we have "apples to apples" comparisons when using benchmarks or other hospitals' performance as the basis for assessment. The measurement techniques and structures should be the same for valid and reliable comparisons.*

These are just a few examples of pitfalls in measurement. How do you prevent and correct them in your hospital? Typically, the PI director and/or employees in that department are the "internal consultants" for the hospital in measurement. They should teach employees about PI and encourage them to "keep it simple" and develop highly focused goals and measures.

The PI director and his or her staff, if any, should receive basic education in quality data collection and assessment (see Figure 6.7) so that they are comfortable with the primary problems and solutions for effective data management.

Developing reliable data collection methods

Even a well-thought-out plan for data collection can break down when pencil touches paper to record the data. Often, problems occur because staff members don't understand the specific definitions of data they are supposed to capture, or because the written tools are ambiguous, or because they wish to sabotage the data.

For example, if a check sheet is developed to evaluate whether patient records indicate that patients were told the risks and benefits of a blood transfusion, the sheet might have a column labeled "risks explained?" This is a relatively unclear question as it stands. Somewhere on the page, the specific risks should be listed that, according to hospital policy, should have been explained to the patient. It may be that your hospital is particularly interested in ensuring that the risk of a transfusion reaction has been correctly and clearly explained. In that case, the check sheet should highlight that specific question. On the other hand, perhaps you want to ensure that all risks have been explained; staff members should know exactly what you are looking for, and the sheet needs to be set up so that they can highlight what was and what was not documented in accordance with policy.

Sabotage is a real problem with data collection, and it is not necessarily a problem that arises only with sinister intent or among poorly performing employees. It is very possible for staff to bias data in innumerable ways, and it is not always feasible to design data collection to prevent sabotage. It is important to be cognizant of the risks and have means to sample or audit the data, test the data for reasonableness, use multiple data collectors, and work constantly to ensure that staff members understand and support the effort for which data are being collected. This is a human process that depends on human beings' cooperation and commitment to improvement, and it has to be performed in a "PI" culture.

As an example, consider the simple waiting time log sheet. If staff members know that their individual and collective performance reviews depend on shorter waiting times, what could be more natural than "skimming" a few minutes off the time they write on the log sheet? We all hope that we can work constructively with our employees to help them feel a part of the improvement process and to help them understand how counterproductive such "shading" of the data would be, but it is the wiser course to also monitor the data and ensure that the integrity of people and information is maintained. Furthermore, if staff members are sabotaging data, your discovery of this will be essential to enable you to help allay their concerns or address their fears before the PI initiative can move forward.

A more complex example arises when staff members gather data that they know will be used to assess productivity and cost-effectiveness. One example is in patient acuity systems, often used in nursing areas to determine the workload represented by a group of patients. Some of the measures typically used are objective and can be audited (e.g., "patient is bedridden" or "patient has been placed on fall precautions"). Other measures, such as "assistance to toilet" or "special psychological and teaching needs," may be interpreted differently among staff members and may be subject to manipulation. In these instances, it may be helpful to look at the use of these subjective ratings among different staff members. If a certain staff member always seems to think that patients have special needs, and others list this characteristic for only a small proportion of patients, then there may be a problem with interpretation or manipulation.

In summary, we all should remember the old "garbage in, garbage out" rule. It is only prudent to take a hard look at specific data collected by staff members, particularly those entered manually, which are hard to audit, subject to interpretation and judgment, and likely to be perceived by staff as potentially threatening. The quality of the data is so important for decision making that this is worth some time and energy.

Evaluating data

If you have ensured that the data being collected is focused and reasonably valid, the next challenge is to make sense of the data. The single most frequent question about data is "have we really changed our performance?" This is why the JCAHO recommends the use of statistical process control (SPC) as a technique. It is relatively easy to compute and implement, is pertinent to a wide range of processes (though not all), and can be set up with simple personal computing tools. It can answer the question of whether a meaningful shift in performance has occurred. (The Bibliography section in this book offers good sources on SPC.)

Other statistical tools can be useful as well. A simple student's T-test to evaluate the significance of a change in means is commonly used and relatively easy to set up. Measures of dispersion, such as the standard deviation and coefficient of variation, can be computed using a standard spreadsheet, and they can show whether performance is becoming more consistent. Common computer programs that will help you with these tasks include Microsoft Excel or Lotus spreadsheet software for the basics and, if needed, SPSS or SAS for more sophisticated statistics.

When your hospital chooses which comparative performance databases it will join (for the PI and information management standards, see Chapters 1, 2, and 3), you may wish to seek a comparative database that offers some statistical information about your performance compared to the benchmark or comparison group (many of these comparative systems provide this). For instance, major patient satisfaction comparative databases provide information on (1) your hospital's mean scores compared to those of a peer group, (2) whether these means are statistically different from the peer group mean, (3) whether they've improved or declined significantly over time, (4) where your score falls as a percentile among the group, and perhaps (5) correlation coefficients among the survey items to help you understand what is important to patients.

Establishing performance improvement training programs

Every hospital has its own training culture. Some hospitals do a lot of training in-house and may even have their own "university" or "school" set up for a wide variety of training programs. Others tend to purchase training outside and send staff to seminars. For many, budgets may not have extensive resources for travel and seminars, and they may rely on books and journals to keep them current (see Bibliography for a list of suggested readings).

In developing training, one key is to establish targeted programs for each different group with its own unique needs, such as

- Leader/manager training (including medical leaders)
- New employee training/orientation
- Team training
- Statistical training

Leader and manager training

As noted before, all new managers and medical staff leaders must be oriented to the hospital's PI philosophy and methodology. This will ensure that they understand both their responsibility and accountability in the PI program and which support resources are available to them.

Chapter 6

In addition, this sort of training fulfills a number of the JCAHO's leadership, medical staff, human resources, information management, and PI requirements. Therefore, you should be sure to document all training activities, perhaps by simply listing who received what training and outlining the corresponding orientation program.

Training and orientation of new employees

It is important for JCAHO compliance that some exposure to PI principles be offered to every employee in the hospital. Surveyors will ask what proportion of hospital employees have been "trained" in the methodology and priorities for PI in the hospital. The definition of training is your own, and you will be wise to ensure that you can respond that 100% of the work force is exposed to the concepts.

One approach is to conduct a brief introductory session at new employee orientation; although this is challenging, considering the varied audience, it can be successful (Figure 6.9 contains a model program and Figure 6.10 provides a helpful exercise designed to teach staff about PI).

Another approach is to ensure that all managers conduct some formal PI training each year, documenting attendance and curriculum, perhaps in the context of staff meetings. Some organizations have gone further and have mandated attendance of the entire work force at formal PI training sessions, an expensive initiative whose justification certainly will depend on productive use of the information provided. These approaches can also, of course, be combined and used appropriately for different areas of the hospital.

Team training

See Chapter 7 for an in-depth review of team formation and training needs. It is important that teams receive appropriate training to increase their ability to produce successful outcomes.

Statistical training

Individuals, departments, or teams that will be required to design new measures must be trained on the basics of reliable data collection, analysis, and interpretation. This training may be incorporated into new manager orientation and team workshops, or both.

Remember to document all employee training sessions in measurement and statistics. This will help you demonstrate compliance with the JCAHO's human resources and information management standards.

Monitoring implementation of performance improvement throughout the hospital

Broadly speaking, the hospital's PI director is responsible for monitoring all aspects of PI through the cycle. For example, you should evaluate each department's compliance with the hospital's policies and standards for meetings, minutes, and data collection and analysis; you should check on each team's progress and ensure that each makes reports to sponsoring management or committees as scheduled; and you should manage the hospital's annual self-assessment process (see Chapter 11).

On a day-to-day basis, it's the quality department's responsibility to monitor the progress of all departments conducting measurements and ensure that the measurements are taken and

FIGURE 6.9

Agenda for performance improvement orientation of new employees

Objectives
Participants in this session will learn to
- Identify the major customer groups served by the hospital
- Recognize that quality is defined by the customer
- Describe our hospital's definition of quality
- Understand the importance of patient and customer satisfaction and PI and how they can further both these ideals

Hands-On Introduction to Quality
"The red card game" (Figure 6.10 gives a description)

Discussion
What is quality?
Who decides whether we deliver quality?
- Customers judge quality
- Who are our customers?
  - Patients
  - Family members
  - Insurance payers
  - Physicians
  - Community
  - Government/accreditation agencies
  - Training/research programs
  - One another!

How do you know what the customer wants?
Ask, don't assume; think about customers' underlying needs.

How do you know if you are meeting customer needs?
Ask, and then measure.

What's even better than correcting a problem for a customer?
Prevention and continuous improvement.

Who is responsible for quality?
Everyone serves the patient ultimately.

What is quality at our hospital?
What each employee must do.

What will you do?

---

interpreted correctly. In addition, this department should occasionally evaluate the size of the samples for analysis, the evidence that a trend was statistically meaningful, the possibility that unconsidered external factors drove the observed change in performance, and so on. Thoughtful review of departments' quality reports is an important component of the quality department's task and is important to ensure that you provide good feedback to managers to help them enhance their own skills in PI.

Chapter 6

FIGURE 6.10

The "red card game" leader guide

This game was created based on the principles taught by W. Edwards Deming in the famous "red bead experiment." The goals are to teach (in approximately 5 minutes) the basic PI principle that quality depends on systems and the key point that we are each part of a system. The experiment is low-cost and portable. Conduct this during your new employee PI training sessions (see Figure 6.8).

This exercise will teach staff the following lessons:

- We are all part of complex systems.
- We depend on one another.
- When we fail, or when the outcome is not as we wish, we should examine the system to see where it may be breaking down.
- Blaming colleagues obscures underlying systems issues.
- The role of every worker is to contribute ideas about possible underlying systems problems in a constructive process.
- The role of management is to improve systems to make optimum use of workers' talents and energy.

Directions:
Flip through a standard deck of playing cards and select five "red" cards (i.e., diamonds or hearts) and five "black" cards (i.e., spades or clubs). Set the remaining cards aside. Organize the ten cards into two piles, and sequence them face down in the following order:

Deck 1	Deck 2
(top of pile)	(top of pile)
1. Red card	1. Black card
2. Black card	2. Black card
3. Red card	3. Red card
4. Red card	4. Black card
5. Red card	5. Black card

Ask for two volunteers from your training session. Hand one volunteer "Deck 1" and tell him that he is a nurse. Hand the second volunteer "Deck 2" and tell her that she is a food service employee. Ask each volunteer to select a "patient" from the crowd.

Announce that the correct meal and the correct medication are denoted by black cards. Instruct the volunteers to either "administer the medication" or "give the patient a meal tray" by handing their respective "patients" a card from the top of the decks they are holding. The volunteers should not look at the cards.

Instruct the "patients" to hold up their meal/medication cards. Praise the "food service employee" for her competence. Express dramatic disappointment with the "nurse," and patiently explain to him that "black" is the right medication. Assure him that the patient suffered no ill effects from the "medication error," and encourage him to try harder tomorrow.

Go through another round, stating that it is now "tomorrow." Praise the food service employee again, and express delight that the nurse "got the message from our little chat yesterday." Make a big deal about her apparent improvement in response to your wonderful management coaching.

Third round: Pretend to be shocked at the slip in the food service employee's performance; ask her if she had a bad night and didn't get any rest or forgot the hospital's performance standards. Remind her that

FIGURE 6.10 (cont'd)

> black is the right meal, give her a pat on the shoulder, and suggest that tomorrow will be another day. Chastise the nurse for his poor performance, expressing sorrow and disappointment that he wasn't able to sustain yesterday's improved performance.
>
> Fourth round: Express happiness that the food service employee has returned to "full performance" and that, again, your terrific management skills and coaching were effective. Suggest to the nurse that we might need to talk about putting him on probation.
>
> Fifth round: If time permits, conduct a fifth round. You can discuss disciplinary action for the nurse and a possible promotion for the food service worker.
>
> **Discussion:**
> Lots of giggles and uncomfortable laughter always accompany this exercise. Always give the "victims" the first chance to discuss the game. Ask them both how they felt during the game, and try to elicit feelings of helplessness, frustration, and fear.
>
> Ask the group at large why they think you held this exercise during a discussion of quality and performance. Major themes that are usually discussed are "I'm part of a system," "I depend on my co-workers," I don't always control my own performance," and so on.
>
> Sometimes employees will start on a theme of "blaming" the department that assembled the meal trays or medications. Steer them toward thinking about those departments as they did the "victims." For example, what if the kitchen didn't have the right meal orders in front of them when they assembled the trays? What if the pharmacy had the wrong information or items were out of place?

Reprinted by permission of Northwestern Memorial Hospital, Chicago, IL.

Other responsibilities of performance improvement directors

Although not directly related to JCAHO compliance, a few other common responsibilities of PI directors are drawing increasing concern and do have potential to enhance compliance while meeting other goals as well. These include responding to managed care requests for quality information and interfacing with peer review organizations in their new "PI" role.

Responding to managed care requests for information

It is more and more common for managed care contracts to request information about quality measures. Every company has its own unique data elements of interest, and common definitions of terms have not yet emerged. Thus, responding to these inquiries can be labor intensive and even risky if your hospital is using a definition (e.g., of nosocomial infections) that is more stringent than most. Common data requests may include requests for information on

- Patient satisfaction
- Infection rates
- Mortality rates, perhaps overall or for individual diagnoses or DRGs

- "Complications" or "adverse event" rates (often only vaguely defined)
- Lengths of stay for specific diagnoses and/or DRGs
- Your quality program, perhaps including a specific request for minutes of quality meetings

It is beyond the scope of this book to address the many issues involved in the decision about whether to provide all of the information managed care organizations request. From the quality professional's point of view, it is imperative that the complexity of these requests and the problems associated with their typical vagueness be fully recognized. It would be wise to develop and adopt through your quality committee a specific policy on what data may be disclosed, who may disclose it, and what approval process is required to disclose additional data items. Legal advice will be needed as well.

From a JCAHO point of view, such a policy will be pertinent to compliance with information management standards and potentially with patients' rights standards. Allowing disclosure on condition that you receive comparative reports back from the managed care organization may help you to comply with information management and PI standards related to benchmarking and comparative data analysis.

Interfacing with peer review organizations

In the past, an important role for quality department staff was to interact with the Medicare peer review organization (PRO) staff regarding negative findings the PRO might issue on an individual patient's care. This function does still continue, though it is much less common than in the 1980s.

Contemporary PRO focus has shifted to collaborative projects with hospitals related to core clinical processes. Although still new, this revised focus has also changed the ways in which quality professionals work with the PRO. More often now, the quality department (1) evaluates projects proposed by the PRO to determine if there is opportunity for learning and benchmarking important processes, (2) recommends participation to the quality oversight committee, (3) implements the project through data collection, (4) attends meetings to share data with other hospitals, and (5) brings final conclusions of the project back to the hospital for evaluation of their implications for changing processes there. Examples may include studies of the cardiac bypass clinical pathway, pneumonia diagnosis and treatment, and prevention of decubitus ulcers.

This type of collaboration is another area with rich possibilities for JCAHO compliance in comparative and benchmarked data analysis (e.g., information management and PI standards) as well as leadership standards related to improving the health of the community.

Chapter 7

Working Successfully with Performance Improvement Teams

Working in multidisciplinary teams is hard work, mainly because teams transcend traditional management control systems and rely on solid data, consensus processes, creativity, and shared values and goals to succeed. They require individual team members to be willing to relinquish individual rewards in favor of benefit to the customer and the hospital.

Overseeing the work of multidisciplinary teams and integrating them into individual departments' goals, quality plans, and priorities is also a significant challenge for hospital leaders. Multidisciplinary teams do not readily elicit the level of commitment and energy that traditional intradepartmental improvement efforts do, and it takes a skillful person to overcome these roadblocks. It is generally easier to make changes in a single department, where one manager controls all the available resources and rewards, than to encourage a collection of departments to work together on an issue that no one person directly controls. For example, every department involved in "reducing waiting time for an inpatient admission" is no doubt busy and believes itself admirably productive and successful. Moreover, it may be hard to encourage each individual department to agree on a single goal toward which to work.

In addition, the more complex the team and the process under study, the greater the likelihood you'll contend with intentional or unintentional sabotage because of a lack of commitment, fear of change, challenge to authority, or withholding of resources. For example, the nursing staff may not want to accept inpatient admissions during shift changes, even if not doing so slows the system. Housekeeping may not want to "float" to clean rooms on other floors, even if this is needed, because it may appear to reduce efficiency and productivity in that department. Admitting may simply want to conduct clear-cut measurements that focus on their own small piece of the process and then be left alone.

Nevertheless, teamwork is the only way to resolve the biggest process problems that face healthcare—that is to say, most of the problems that matter—and therefore it is important that you learn how to work with teams and guide them to success. Read through this chapter for practical information on how best to charter, support, and document the work of your Performance Improvement (PI) teams. You'll learn how to guide your PI teams to success and demonstrate compliance with the Joint Commission on Accreditation of Healthcare Organizations' (JCAHO's) requirements.

Chapter 7

When do you need a performance improvement team?

Most hospitals use PI teams to help them implement multidisciplinary PI action plans. Complex, multidisciplinary processes require multiple perspectives and considerable collaboration and creativity for improvement, and teams are an optimal approach. In addition, the JCAHO requires you to implement multidisciplinary and multidepartmental improvement efforts, and using PI teams will help you meet that requirement.

Your hospital-wide PI plan, described in Chapter 8, outlines your approach to your "big-picture" goals for PI this year, such as reducing infection rates, improving radiology turn-around times, or shortening lengths of stay for a particular procedure. For most of these projects, you will most definitely need to charter PI teams to tackle the project. But smaller, departmental projects might be best handled by a department manager.

As you try to decide whether an improvement project warrants a PI team, you should consider one key issue: Do you really know how to perform this process effectively and efficiently for the customer? If you do, then you just need "enforcement" or management processes put in place to help ensure that staff perform the procedure correctly. Examples of such an enforcement process might be quality indicators for hand washing or timely medication charting. Processes that are good candidates for this monitoring tend to be "smaller" processes, performed by one person or a small group within a department without extensive dependence on others.

If not, and the process in question is a priority for your customers and your hospital (see Chapter 8), then you should charter a team to reconsider the process and determine whether there is a better way to perform it to meet the needs of the customer.

Selecting a performance improvement team model

Once you've decided that you do indeed need a PI team to handle an improvement project, you should select the best "PI team model" for your team. You may choose any of the following PI team models, depending on the type of problem you are trying to correct and the amount of human and financial resources at your disposal:

- A coached team
- A self-directed team
- A manager-directed team
- A narrowly focused team

Coached team
This model calls for a "coach" or "facilitator" to oversee all of the team's efforts. Somewhat widely used in industry, this model is less common in healthcare, where there are few trained coaches in a given hospital.

The coach works with the designated team leader, often behind the scenes, to

- Ensure that the team understands how to use the hospital's PI model and work as a team
- Teach the team members data management techniques or suggest useful data collection and analysis methods

- Work with the team's leader to overcome interpersonal conflicts on the team or identify when it might be a good time for senior managers to clarify the team's charter and parameters
- Edit the team's results to ensure that they follow the hospital's standard for presentations

For particularly high-risk and high-potential-benefit teams, a "coach" model may be a worthwhile investment. The greatest advantage of the coach model is that each team will have professional, objective counseling all the way through its efforts and can likely produce results more quickly. The greatest disadvantage, interestingly, is that the coach can become an authority figure who both detracts from the team leader's authority and, even more problematically, can become a substitute for the senior managers who need ultimately to review and accept the team's work.

Self-directed team

The term *self-directed team* has come to mean a work group that works together over a long period to make an improvement, such as a group of nurses, physicians, dietitians, pharmacists, and support personnel, who are all working together to improve care in a patient care unit. These team members are trained by a manager but remain independent of the trainer and make their own decisions.

The greatest risks of using this model are that the team may get bogged down by a lack of authority or that a single, authoritative individual may take over the entire group. This does not mean that the team should be leaderless; on the contrary, a good leader is essential and should make a genuine effort to bring all of the team members' ideas together. If the members of the team are able to see each other as equal in authority in the organization and if the team shares a commitment to the goal of the team, a self-directed model may be effective.

Manager-directed team

In many hospitals, managers of the areas that are going to be improved are chosen as PI team leaders and direct the work of their PI teams. This "manager-directed model" can work very well if the process in question is self-contained within the department and the manager in question has good facilitation skills.

The primary pitfall for such an effort arises when the manager is perceived by staff to have a predetermined agenda and outcome, and staff are unwilling or unable to participate fully and creatively in the improvement process. For example, if a manager has conceptually redesigned the transportation dispatch process and performance standards, it will not be productive to form a PI team to improve the process; the manager already knows what he or she wants to accomplish. In this instance, the manager should be using change-management tools rather than PI tools to bring the employees into consonance with his or her vision of the new process.

On the other hand, if the manager genuinely wants a creative and open process to evaluate different alternatives and consider new approaches, a team can work well. The manager can serve as team leader as long as the team effort has integrity and the manager's role as the authority in the department does not inhibit the team's measurements, assessment, and improvements.

A common variation of a manager-directed team is for two managers to co-lead a team that involves both of their departments. This can certainly work if both managers are genuinely

Chapter 7

open to the work of the team, both have good facilitation skills, and the managers' authority roles will not stifle the creativity and honesty of team members. In addition, these teams may need to do some work to build relationships across departmental lines to foster trust and openness among staff who may have had past problems with each other.

Narrowly focused team

Most hospitals end up establishing narrowly focused task teams to tackle their improvement projects. Because of its relatively low cost and relative ease of startup, this model remains the most common and practical one for most PI teams.

Generally, these teams are led by someone who has the ability to keep a group on target. They are also supported by the hospital, which provides data management expertise, facilitation help, training for all members of the team, solid management support, and commitment to keep the team on track.

The great advantage of these narrowly focused teams is that they can be held to relatively short lives, perhaps 3–6 months, which reduces the danger of burnout and stalemates.

The risk is that without professional facilitation (the coach model) or long-term planned interdependence (the self-directed team approach), the group may flounder because of a lack of commitment or familiarity with the technical tools of PI. Selecting and training a capable leader can reduce these risks.

Choosing performance improvement team members and chartering the team

You should select your PI team members carefully. Ideally, you'll choose individuals who have first-hand knowledge of the process you're trying to improve, since these individuals should be able to pinpoint what works and what doesn't and can offer suggestions on how to make improvements. For example, individuals from the housekeeping, admitting, nursing, and transportation departments would be ideal members of a PI team trying to reduce time from admission to an inpatient bed.

There is considerable disagreement in PI literature about whom to place on a PI team. If you compose the team solely of managers, your members will have the authority to commit money and resources to a problem. If you compose your team solely of front-line staff who perform the process every day, you'll gain invaluable data and experience in what does and does not work in the process. Generally, a combination works best. This way you'll have both the authority and the knowledge of the process you need to solve the problem.

Chartering the PI team should be done formally. A sample team charter is shown in Figure 7.1. The charter should include

- A description of the process to be improved
- A list of all the PI team members
- The team's goals
- The team's schedule or timeline
- A reference to the particular JCAHO functions and dimensions the team will work to improve

FIGURE 7.1

Sample performance improvement team charter

Directions: This charter should be completed by the PI team's sponsor on formation of a PI team to ensure that both the team and its sponsor are on the same track and understand exactly what needs to be done.

Process we want to improve:

_____

_____

Primary customers:

_____

_____

Secondary customers:

_____

_____

	Name	**Department**	**Phone**
Team sponsor:			
Team leader:			
Team members:			

Why is this improvement important to the hospital and its customers at this time?

_____

_____

Chapter 7

FIGURE 7.1 (cont'd)

How is this improvement linked to the hospital's strategic plan and to all applicable departments' missions and goals?
_____
_____

Tentative timetable for completing the team's work:
_____
_____

Improvement project can be classified in these JCAHO terms: (Chapter 10 provides a detailed discussion of these requirements.)

Dimensions of performance	**JCAHO functions**
❑ Efficacy	❑ Patient rights and organization ethics
❑ Appropriateness	❑ Assessment of patients
❑ Availability	❑ Care of patients
❑ Timeliness	❑ Patient and family education
❑ Effectiveness	❑ Continuum of care
❑ Continuity of care	❑ Improving organizational performance
❑ Safety	❑ Leadership
❑ Efficiency	❑ Management of the environment of care
❑ Respect/caring	❑ Management of human resources
	❑ Management of information
	❑ Surveillance, prevention, and control of infection

The team will refer to this document repeatedly to ensure that it's on track. And, of course, this charter will clearly document your PI team's goals for JCAHO surveyors.

Training task teams on the performance improvement model

Although some organizations invest in quality and process improvement training for 100% of staff, others opt to hold "just in time" training workshops for teams as they are formed. An

FIGURE 7.2

Outline of a "just in time" performance improvement training workshop

"Just in time" PI training sessions are designed to teach PI team members how to work with the hospital's chosen PI model to implement improvements. This session should take no longer than one-half a day and should be led by someone very experienced in PI, such as the hospital's PI director or the PI team's sponsor.

This session will teach PI teams how to

- Develop a written mission statement that elaborates on its initial team charter
- Develop a graphic logo or picture that embodies the team's identity
- Determine exactly who are the customers of the process in question and what their needs are
- Flow-chart the current process
- Create a list of data collection tasks and measurements the team should conduct to reach conclusions about the nature of the current process and customer perceptions of it
- Gather comparative data and benchmarks to determine how the process is conducted at other organizations
- Establish an action plan and assign responsibility and schedules for certain data collection and research tasks
- Set a meeting schedule for the next 6–12 weeks, with defined responsibilities for administrative tasks and minute-taking
- Secure the team's sponsor's formal approval of the proposed schedule and action plan

Figure 7.3 provides a sample agenda for such a session.

---

outline and sample agenda of one "just in time" workshop, which focuses on giving the team a jump-start on its effort, are shown in Figures 7.2 and 7.3.

These "just in time" workshops should teach the teams how to use the hospital's PI model. For example, a workshop should teach the team

- How to draft up its mission, objectives, flow diagram, and work plan
- The basics of data management

Usually, these issues are covered in one half-day session. In addition, you might consider holding a "how to lead a team" workshop, focusing on the life cycles of teams and work groups, team facilitation skills, the differences between a team and a formal organizational unit with designated authority, and task planning (Figure 7.4 provides an outline of such a session).

Before the team begins to investigate its assigned issue, you should ensure that each member has a full understanding of the process under study and the problem that led to the team's charter. For example, the team may have been presented with an objective (e.g., reduce the infection rate for this procedure to 4%) or may have been presented with an opportunity for further exploration (e.g., compare our infection rate for this procedure to that of similar hospitals and determine a reasonable goal for reduction). Whatever the issue may be, you should ensure that the team fully understands the history of the problem.

FIGURE 7.3

Sample "just in time" performance improvement training workshop agenda

12:00 p.m.	**Introductions**
	The PI process and the PI team
	• Understanding the team charter
	• Developing a team identity
12:30 p.m.	**How we work together as a team**
	• Our process improvement model
	• Creating team norms
	• Examining team roles and stages
1:00 p.m.	**How we define quality**
	• Quality overview
	• Defining customer needs
1:25 p.m.	**Break**
1:30 p.m.	**What we're here to do**
	• Developing a team mission statement
1:50 p.m.	**Analysis of the process**
	• Introduction to flow charting
	• Flow-charting the process
	• Other analytical tools
3:15 p.m.	**Break**
3:20 p.m.	**The next steps**
	• Action planning
	• Conducting effective team meetings
4:00 p.m.	**Concluding remarks and questions**
4:30 p.m.	**Adjournment**

Supporting your performance improvement teams

Regardless of whether you have a coached team, self-directed team, manager-directed team, or narrowly focused team, you will need to provide it with continuous support. Most likely, your teams will need you to

- Coach them through inevitable interpersonal issues
- Suggest creative new approaches to problems when the team stalemates

FIGURE 7.4

Outline of a "how to lead a performance improvement team" workshop

Often, it's worth the time to hold a "how to lead a team" workshop for PI team leaders. This workshop should focus on the life cycles of teams and work groups, team facilitation skills, the differences between a team and a formal organizational unit with designated authority, and task planning. An agenda for such a session follows.

WORKSHOP AGENDA

Introduction
- The differences between work groups and teams
- What you want from this session

The ideal team and team leader
- Learning leadership techniques, such as brainstorming and consensus building

How teams function
- Learning how teams work through role play, observation, and discussion

Communication skills to encourage participation and involvement
- Team communication patterns

Team stages (forming, storming, norming, performing)
- The leader's role at each stage

Conducting meetings
- What makes a meeting productive or unproductive?
- Learning how to plan, facilitate, and conduct such a meeting.
- Developing an agenda.
- Focusing on a meeting.
- Concluding a meeting, establishing action plans, and obtaining feedback.

- Help collect and analyze data
- Identify benchmarks
- Produce concise and compelling reports and recommendations
- Navigate departmental boundaries
- Help develop constructive new processes

Typically, these activities fall to the quality resource department, but they may be shared with other areas, such as organization development, management engineering, or even a medical library.

FIGURE 7.5

Common performance improvement tools

Each PI team in your hospital will use a number of PI tools to help them evaluate processes and determine what improvements should be made. This table of common tools is intended to focus on generic analysis tools that can be useful to teams but are often overlooked, underutilized, or misused due to unfamiliarity. For more information on these tools, refer to the Bibliography section of this book for a listing of excellent sources for more information. Each tool has been mapped to the JCAHO's "Plan, Design, Measure, Assess, Improve" system to let you know at what stage you can use each tool.

Common tools	Plan	Design	Measure	Assess	Improve
Focus groups, interviews, surveys of opinion/perception	✓		✓		
Reviews of complaints, incident reports, litigation, etc.	✓		✓		
Chart reviews, checklists to evaluate whether past performance has incorporated all desired elements	✓		✓		
Literature reviews, benchmark research	✓	✓			
Analysis of historical performance and trends on quality measures (often using run charts and/or control charts, if appropriate to the type of data)	✓	✓	✓	✓	
Brainstorming to identify potential sources of performance problems	✓			✓	
Scatter diagrams to see relationships among quantitative factors	✓		✓	✓	
Flow-charting to see the process and its problems, delays, etc.	✓	✓		✓	
Affinity diagrams to bring brainstormed ideas into thematic units	✓			✓	
Force field analysis to assess the importance of variables in driving or constraining performance	✓			✓	
Cause-and-effect ("fishbone" or Ishikawa) diagram to sort out potential process problems into categories and groups	✓			✓	
Histogram and Pareto charts to focus on the "vital few" factors that affect performance and to set aside the "trivial many" factors that obscure issues	✓		✓	✓	
Nominal group technique to reach consensus on the relative importance of issues (also multivoting)	✓	✓		✓	✓

FIGURE 7.5 (cont'd)

Common tools	Plan	Design	Measure	Assess	Improve
Prioritization matrix to select best approaches through systematically weighting factors and comparing options on these weighted factors	✓	✓			✓
Design of experiments (DOE) methods of testing interventions and process changes systematically		✓	✓	✓	
Quality function deployment to select priorities systematically	✓	✓			
Gant chart to plan the team's work over time and keep momentum going	✓	✓	✓	✓	✓

Guiding performance improvement teams through the "Plan, Design, Measure, Assess, and Improve" process

You'll also need to guide each PI team through the entire improvement process—planning, designing, measuring, assessing, and improving. Each team member will have been educated on your hospitals' PI model and PI process during annual quality training sessions or "just in time" training sessions, but you'll need to be available to ensure that each person understands how to put this theory into practice.

Read through the following sections to learn just what is expected of a PI team throughout the improvement process. Also see Figure 7.5 for a list of PI tools teams may use throughout this process.

Plan

During this phase, the PI team defines its purpose, such as "this team will improve medication administration," and plans out exactly what it will need to do to accomplish that goal, such as studying the medication administration process, developing and analyzing measures, and setting goals for improvement, such as "medication errors related to timeliness will be reduced to x per 10,000 patient doses."

As the team develops its plan, it should

- Consider the needs of patients, staff, and other employees directly and indirectly involved in the process
- Evaluate community performance standards if available and pertinent
- Document and evaluate the current processes in place, perhaps using flow charts or similar techniques
- Develop a work plan, which includes meeting schedules, and perhaps a Gant chart of project steps
- Establish who will take minutes, who will send mailings, who will arrange for conference rooms, and so on

FIGURE 7.6

Performance improvement team action plans

Every PI team should develop action plans that describe the actions the team must take and when each will be accomplished. The action plan is a very useful tool that can help keep the team on track, and it will constantly evolve as the work progresses.

Action plans should be written up and included with the minutes of every team meeting. A discussion of the progress of the action plan and any necessary modifications should be the beginning and ending agenda topics of every meeting. This discipline will keep the team as productive as possible.

Sample action plan for team working on admission time from the emergency department

What	Who	When	Cost/resources
Measurement phase			
Measure current time to admission from ED	Jane	March 1	8 hours/week with help from quality committee staff
Call 10 other emergency departments for their measure	Thomas	March 1	10 hours
Develop comparative graph report on ED time	Sally	March 15	5 hours
Assessment phase			
Special meeting to analyze the results	Team	March 16	2 hours
Write up our findings to date and review with quality committee	Alice and team	March 23	8 hours
Focus groups with patients to establish new target	Marketing and team	April 15	20 hours

Design

In the design phase, the team specifically outlines how it will improve the process in question and develops an action plan (Figure 7.6). For example, if the team is working to improve medication administration, it will need to improve staff training, enhance information systems support, make changes to the medication administration record or Kardex as appropriate, and improve communications between nursing and the pharmacy.

The design stage is driven by the planning stage. For example, the team will use what it uncovered in the planning stage to design its improvements. If during the planning phase the team discovered that medication timeliness errors were related to lack of staff awareness and unclear documentation of medication schedules, then the design phase must address those findings (e.g., we will provide staff education to enhance awareness of the importance of timeliness and improve the information system to make the orders clearer).

At this point, the team may also decide to improve other aspects of the process, even if these did not directly contribute to the problem under study; however, the team should be able to define why these changes are in fact improvements, how they believe these changes will be beneficial, and how they intend to measure and assess them.

Measure

After the team has designed the new process, it's ready to pilot-test the process and measure its quality. The measures the team uses should

- Be valid and reliable
- Offer comparisons to outside data or benchmarks, if available
- Be taken with attention to the cost-benefit of data collection (e.g., sampling is adequate but not excessive)

As much as possible, measurement should be "invisible" to those performing the process, both to reduce opportunities for sabotage and to reduce the so-called "Hawthorn effect" in which people perform better simply because they know they are being observed.

Assess

Once all the data is collected, the teams should analyze it, using statistical process control or other valid methodologies. As they review the data, the team members should ask themselves

- Did improvement occur? Was it a statistically reliable change?
- Did improvement occur as much as desired? Are we now in our target range of performance, based on our goal setting and benchmarking?
- What actually changed in the process? Did our design actually get executed accurately?
- What did and did not work in the changed design? (You may get successful results even if portions of the new process are not being performed as you designed them!)
- If the process did not produce sufficient reliable improvement, how can we research the reasons for this?
- If it did produce improvement, do we know specifically what process changes were directly responsible for the improvement?
- Do we have evidence that the improvement will be stable over time and does not depend on constant scrutiny (the so-called Hawthorn effect) for continuation?

Their assessments may also demonstrate the need for more measurements. For example, if you're trying to improve patient satisfaction by reducing wait time, and your assessment indicates that waiting time is down but patient satisfaction has not improved, that indicates that there was something in the patient satisfaction equation that you did not fully understand; you may need to go back and research and study to find out what is missing.

Improve

Once the team's assessments show that the revised process design is indeed producing the desired results, the team should make the new design permanent. For example, the pilot test might be extended to all areas, or it might be ratified through formal policy changes, or

Chapter 7

management may decide that full implementation must be delayed while resources are identified or until training takes place.

Analyzing the performance improvement team's results

After the PI teams have analyzed the process in question and determined whether any improvements should be made, it's up to each team and its sponsor to decide whether the hospital has the time and the resources to implement the changes they recommend.

As you look over their recommendations, you should remember that the JCAHO does not require hospitals to allocate resources to change the level of performance of the process in question; it only requires management to ensure that the undesirable level of performance is fully assessed. For example, if the team's assessment determines that your hospital simply cannot deliver the level of patient satisfaction that the benchmark describes—perhaps you just can't process an admission from the emergency department in 20 minutes!—then quality committee minutes should clearly document the assessment and management's decision to let the issue rest at this time. You may elect to continue to monitor the measure to ensure that it doesn't get worse; or you may decide to move on to other measures that offer some hope for improvement.

It should be emphasized, however, that measurement data that reveals a real and significant risk to patient safety or care should not be ignored. If there are patterns of medication errors, or an increase in patient adverse outcomes, or any measure that reasonably indicates that patient well-being is threatened, JCAHO surveyors will expect to see solid evidence of management commitment to research the problem and address it appropriately and promptly.

Dealing with a team's failure

What if improvement does not occur? What if the team fails? What should you do if a team finds that further improvement is not possible, practical, cost-justified, or perhaps even desirable (e.g., maybe there are unforeseen side effects of a change)?

From a technical and compliance point of view, it is perfectly acceptable to discharge a team that has reached these conclusions, thank them for their work, and document that the process was studied and that the hospital's conclusion is that further investment in this process is not warranted at this time.

From a human point of view, this is a challenge to the relevant managers. You want your PI teams to feel successful and valued. It is a difficult experience to conclude that the team won't be able to improve something that was originally believed to be both important and fixable. To continue to enhance the organization's culture of PI, you will want to work with this group carefully and to honor and respect the hard work the team performed. We all try to do careful work up front, before allocating expensive resources to teams, so such "negative" outcomes are relatively rare in PI. When one does occur, though, it can be used at your quality committees for a positive purpose such as a case study of a team that recognized its limits and made a responsible and appropriate recommendation that respected the hospital's mission and resource limitations.

Part III

Understanding the Performance Improvement Process

Chapter 8

The Blueprint for Success: Developing Your Hospital's Performance Improvement Plan (PI.1)

A hospital's performance improvement (PI) plan is the blueprint for its entire PI program. Just as a hospital is likely to lack strategic focus without a well-thought-out strategic plan, so the PI program is likely to be fragmented and ineffective without a plan that focuses the hospital's energies on common PI priorities and methodologies.

A well-crafted PI plan is crucial to the success of your hospital-wide PI program. It gets everyone speaking a common language and can be a powerful tool for orienting new managers and medical leaders to PI. In addition, this plan often serves as a continuous touchstone or point of reference for the PI oversight committee (see Figure 5.2) throughout the year, helping them to ensure that the PI program is still "on track."

Ironically, given the importance of a PI plan, the Joint Commission on Accreditation of Healthcare Organizations (JCAHO) does not explicitly require hospitals to formally develop one. In fact, the standards include just an offhand reference to PI plans, implying that they "may" be developed, and they do not offer hospitals any advice on what a useful PI plan should include.

This lack of guidance is one of the key reasons that developing a PI plan is one of the most intimidating tasks facing hospitals today. But that doesn't have to be the case. Common sense and a careful reading of the JCAHO's standards can lead you to develop a fully compliant and useful PI plan for your hospital.

Basically, every PI plan should answer at least the following questions:

- How does our mission relate to PI?
- What is our hospital's PI approach or model?
- Who oversees PI in our organization? Who authorizes PI initiatives? Who receives reports, and when, on the progress of key PI initiatives?
- How do we set PI priorities?
- Which resources in the organization will support PI (e.g., a quality department)?
- What are the hospital's immediate and long-term PI goals?

Chapter 8

Read through this chapter to learn how to establish a PI plan that will not only meet JCAHO requirements but will also advance your program's effectiveness overall. As you begin to craft your plan, remember that there is no such thing as a cookie-cutter PI plan that will meet every hospital's needs. Different hospitals have different priorities, and you should tailor your PI plan to your hospital's own goals.

Defining your performance improvement approach

Before you begin to document your PI plan, you must define your hospital's PI approach by (1) selecting a PI model and (2) defining all the hospital leaders' PI responsibilities. Both of these issues are fundamental building blocks for an effective PI program. Typically, a hospital will select its PI model and establish its leaders' PI responsibilities once. After these approaches have been defined, the hospital will need to refine them only every few years. Therefore, it is worth establishing them with care, as you are setting expectations that will support your PI program for years to come.

Selecting a performance improvement model

A PI model is simply a formal description of the thinking and analysis process that your staff will use to consider potential improvement opportunities. PI models are often compared to "the scientific method," and indeed the two look very much alike (e.g., formulate a hypothesis, plan for data collection, test the hypothesis, evaluate the findings, refine the hypothesis, and repeat the cycle). One difference between them is that in PI we are not solely interested in *understanding* a hypothesis. We also want to learn how best to *change* a process once we understand it.

Popular PI models include the JCAHO's own "plan, design, measure, assess, improve" model described in the JCAHO's PI standards, W. Edwards Deming's *"plan, do, check, act"* (PDCA) cycle (derived from Shewhart's "plan, do, study, act" cycle), and Juran's "trilogy" (Figure 8.1 provides comparisons of several popular models to the JCAHO's "plan, design, measure, assess, improve" model). Some hospitals today even use the JCAHO's older "10-step" model with reasonable results. Although each of these models uses different terminology, all of their basic intents are the same. They are designed to help you thoughtfully identify improvement opportunities and correct problems in your organization.

Surveyors will want to see that you consistently use a single PI model throughout your organization. Therefore, your leaders must select one PI model and ensure that every department uses it to implement their PI activities. For example, hospitals cannot allow laboratories to conduct PI activities using W. Edwards Deming's PDCA framework and allow the neurology department to use Juran's "trilogy." Everyone must use the same system.

Your leaders must also ensure that they select a PI model that's easy to implement. For example, a proprietary model designed to be implemented by consultants may be too intricate for a small organization to use efficiently. Or a generic model like Deming's may not offer enough detailed guidance for small hospitals that do not have quality departments to explain the model to staff. Most quality models were not designed specifically for healthcare organizations, and you should be sure to select one that your staff will feel comfortable using. (Figure 8.2 provides a list of issues you should consider before you select a PI model for your hospital.)

Remember that the PI model you select is only a tool. Just because a model tells us to "plan" before we "design" does not mean that the plan will be complete or the design responsive.

FIGURE 8.1

Matching your performance improvement model to the JCAHO's "Plan, Design, Measure, Assess, Improve" model

Occasionally, surveyors have been known to challenge hospitals that use lesser-known PI models simply because they are not using JCAHO terminology. Although it is admittedly easier to communicate with surveyors if you use the JCAHO's own "Plan, Design, Measure, Assess, Improve" (PDMAI) model, there is no reason that you cannot use any reasonable PI model and demonstrate compliance with the PI standards. The key is that you must be able to explain to the surveyors how your PI model compares with the JCAHO's PDMAI.

In the chart below, we've mapped four PI models to the JCAHO's PDMAI model. Mapping models to one another is an inexact science, but the basic principle displayed here is that all models incorporate the same general cyclical approach.

Well before your surveyors arrive at your hospital, map your own PI model to the JCAHO's PDMAI model, and be prepared to explain it to your surveyors on the first day of your survey. The surveyors must understand your PI approach before they even begin to review the hospital's documents or interview staff. Once you've mapped out your system for them, you shouldn't run into any confusion about your PI model or system during their visit.

Comparison of the JCAHO framework to selected other models

Model	Plan	Design	Measure	Assess	Improve
JCAHO 10-step (circa 1992)	1. Assign responsibility	2. Scope of care 3. Important aspects	4. Indicators 5. Thresholds 6. Data collection	7. Evaluate	8. Take action 9. Assess actions 10. Communicate results
Scientific method	Select area of study	Observe what is known Generate hypotheses of causation	Collect data and test hypotheses		Act on findings
Shewhart/Deming PDCA	Plan	Do	Check		Act
FOCUS-PDCA	Find process Organize team Clarify knowledge	Understand cause Select improvement Plan/do	Check		Act

FIGURE 8.2

Selecting a performance improvement model

Before you select a PI model for your organization, consider the following issues:

Q. *Does the hospital already have a common PI language?*

A. If you already have an established PI language, try to find a PI model that coincides with it. Avoid wholesale introduction of a new PI language to your organization; if you must make a significant change, choose your new language carefully and plan to make this a permanent switch. Constant changes in the hospital's "PI lingo" will only serve to confuse employees and hinder the PI process.

Q. *Is the hospital still using the JCAHO 10-step model?*

A. If so, adopting the PDMAI framework will probably be easiest. The hospital obviously has tried to link its program to JCAHO standards in the past, and it will be consistent to use the new framework. JCAHO's own teaching materials include approaches to map the 10-step model to PDMAI, and surveyors will be familiar with the old methodology and are likely to be sympathetic to adjustment issues. It's a competent framework and is likely to be reasonably well received by clinical and professional staff.

Q. *What are the strengths and weaknesses of the hospital's current PI approach?*

A. Ultimately, the decision to enhance or update the hospital's model should be based on a solid understanding of current problems and opportunities. A simple model can be highly effective if staff are educated on the approach and leaders support key improvement opportunities.

Q. *Is the hospital part of a network, an owned system, or a consortium?*

A. If so, consider the possible benefits of sharing a PI framework among all hospitals in the structure. This will facilitate the sharing of best practices and could also make training and support materials portable and less expensive across a larger group.

Q. *Have the hospital's senior leadership or its technical quality leadership had significant success with a particular model at other hospitals?*

A. It may be possible to capitalize on expertise and confidence built at other hospitals. However, no two hospitals have the same culture and history, and prior success is no guarantee of a good fit in a new setting.

Q. *Is the hospital culture highly quantitative and measurement-driven? Or is it more philosophical and mission-driven?*

A. A couple of PI tools, especially the quality function deployment (QFD) technique, are very quantitative. Although these tools may help with certain individual improvement efforts, they should be selected as core methodologies only in hospitals with extensive support resources and with a commitment to teaching the underlying quantitative theory to staff and leaders.

A PI model is simply a set of instructions, and it's up to a hospital's leaders to educate and train all who will use it and to ensure that they implement it correctly.

Defining your leaders' responsibilities

As discussed in Chapter 5, the hospital's leaders drive its PI program. Without their support, your PI efforts cannot succeed. Before you write your PI plan, you should briefly review how you have organized your hospital to perform PI (see Chapter 5 for an overview of which leaders are responsible for which PI activities).

For example, if you've developed a quality oversight committee (see Figure 5.2 on page 74), you should study its charter, including how reports and information will flow to it. You should also note which department heads (i.e., medical staff as well as hospital administrators) are expected to develop and execute PI plans for priorities in their areas. All of this information should be noted in your PI plan. You won't need to discuss it in a great deal of detail, but you will need to "set the stage" to ensure that your readers understand specifically how your organization's leaders participate in PI.

Setting improvement priorities

You should also review your hospital's priority-setting system and determine who is responsible for selecting improvement priorities and how these priorities will be determined. This, too, will later need to be documented in your PI plan. Note that both the PI standards and the leadership (LD) standards require the hospital to establish improvement priorities. We are all familiar with the "Ready, fire, aim!" management style, and to avoid that mistake, you should define the hospital's method of setting priorities. This will ensure that the hospital's energies are thoughtfully channeled and that projects are permitted to come to fruition.

See Chapter 6 for a discussion of how you as PI director can and must stay current on national trends in quality improvement thinking to keep your hospital's priorities appropriate. It is incumbent on the PI function to monitor accreditation, legislative, and regulatory developments that could make an adjustment to PI priorities necessary. Examples of new developments include management of restraints, focus on pain management, the rights of patients for active involvement in decision making regarding their care, the use of clinical practice guidelines, and, of course, the new ORYX and emerging core performance measurement data sets.

Usually, the PI oversight committee is responsible for setting priorities. The group may generate ideas for priorities through brainstorming, review of performance data, or management's and staff's proposals. It can review potential improvement priorities by any method, such as traditional consensus, a highly elaborated numeric point-scoring system, or a formal group process technique, such as multivoting.

It doesn't matter which priority-setting system the committee uses; the keys are that the system is documented in your PI plan, it is systematic and organization-wide, it drives measurement, and it is actually implemented, as evidenced by minutes and other documentation. Hospitals that run into trouble in this area generally have failed to define a prioritization method or have never used the defined method. Remember, it is perfectly fine to define your priority-setting method as simply a group consensus at the quality council once a year or once a quarter, but if you do select such a basic method, you should ensure that the council's discussions and consensus are documented in pertinent minutes.

For some major improvement projects, you may seek the board's approval. The board should look the potential project over and, using the priority-setting criteria listed in its PI plan, determine whether it should be implemented. Corresponding board meeting minutes should note who authorized the project, how this project will advance the hospital's mission, and how it will meet the needs of its patients.

Of course, the threshold at which a particular initiative deserves board attention will vary from hospital to hospital. As an example, you may want board input and review before you bring a costly new drug into the formulary; another hospital may have established procedures for obtaining approval within management and simply informing the board of the decision later. Regardless of the level of management or governance that approves a decision, there should be a reasonably systematic approach to making significant decisions with attention to cost, benefit, and expected performance measures.

And again, what constitutes a "significant" decision varies from hospital to hospital, and it may or may not be spelled out in complete detail. The key for demonstrating JCAHO compliance is not to try to prove that all decisions were processed through an elaborate algorithm incorporating leadership and PI standards but to show how some critical decisions were handled.

Defining the audience for your performance improvement plan

Although JCAHO surveyors will review your PI plan during survey, they are not your plan's primary target audience. They'll simply review your plan to ensure that the hospital complies with all relevant JCAHO standards and adequately plans for and supports PI.

You should write your PI plan for those individuals who will oversee PI in your hospital—your hospital's leaders. All of these leaders, from senior managers to middle and first-line managers, should use the plan to help them define their own PI strategies and goals. Therefore, it's your responsibility to ensure that the plan is clearly written and understood by its entire audience. For example, your plan should give managers guidance on how to implement PI initiatives in both clinical departments, such as nursing or respiratory therapy, and nonclinical departments, such as security, information systems, patient escort, and accounting.

All new managers who will be responsible for PI in some capacity should be required to review this plan to introduce them to your PI program. The plan should be accessible and clear to those who are new to your hospital. It tells them how they fit in, what their role in the hospital's performance program is, and how PI is linked to their job descriptions (e.g., managers should monitor, manage, and improve performance in their area of responsibility).

Developing the performance improvement plan

Once you've defined your PI approach, set your improvement priorities, and defined your audience, you are ready to document your PI plan.

Typically, it will take the quality resources manager several weeks to develop a final PI plan. During this time, this individual will be responsible for

- Gathering background information
- Writing the plan
- Obtaining key leaders' approval

Gathering background information
The hospital's PI plan must be fully integrated with other key hospital-wide plans, such as your leadership plan, and goal setting in the hospital. As emphasized in Chapter 5, effective

and JCAHO-compliant PI activities must be developed in sync with the hospital's strategic and operating priorities for the year, or you will never achieve real improvements that are meaningful to your patients and community.

Before you sit down to document your PI plan, you should review

- Governing body bylaws, which describe the board's accountability for quality and performance
- Medical staff bylaws, which describe the specific responsibilities of medical staff leaders for PI
- The hospital's strategic plan, which will influence your mission description and how you draft the annual PI goals
- The hospital's chosen PI model (e.g., "plan, design, measure, assess, improve" or PDCA), which will be briefly described in the plan
- The hospital's governance structure and committee structures for PI, including committee charters and membership, so that you can briefly summarize them in the plan
- Prior versions of the PI plan
- Meeting minutes documenting suggested improvements to the PI plan and the hospital's current and future improvement priorities

All of these pieces of information will give you the background you need on the hospital's PI program to develop a useful PI plan.

Writing the performance improvement plan

No two PI plans are identical. It's up to you to decide how best to organize the plan to meet your hospital's needs. Each hospital's PI plan reflects its own planning style, speaks effectively to its target audience, and usefully educates its leaders about PI. For example, some successful PI plans that have passed JCAHO review have consisted of just a couple of pages of narrative and an organization chart showing committee responsibilities and relationships, while others have been 40 pages long, containing detailed narrative descriptions of committee functions and confidentiality protections.

But no matter how long or detailed your PI plan is, it must touch on some basic issues. Read through the following sections to learn what key elements must be included in your PI plan and how you should approach each one. Figure 8.3 provides a sample PI plan.

Mission, definition, and goals of the quality program

It is a good idea to "ground" your PI plan with a brief restatement of the hospital's mission, values, vision, and strategic planning goals, because the JCAHO requires you to formally and substantively link the hospital's goals to its PI program. This is also an excellent way to set the stage for an integrated thinking process and to effectively remind your internal audience (i.e., management and medical leadership) that "we don't just do PI because of JCAHO, we do it because it meaningfully supports our mission and our future."

You should also briefly explain how PI is expected to advance the hospital's mission. A sentence or two is sufficient. The goals of the quality program listed here should be broad and general, such as "to improve the care and service rendered to patients and other customers" or "to fulfill our hospital mission." This is not the place to list this year's specific PI goals.

FIGURE 8.3

Northwestern Memorial Hospital's performance improvement plan outline

I. Plan objectives
The PI plan's mission, goals, and purpose

II. Scope
A brief summary of hospital services, including home health agencies, outpatient clinics, and owned physician groups

III. Performance improvement priorities
1. Key quality goals
2. Process for revising priorities
3. Process for routine monitoring, evaluation, and improvement

   Be sure to note that all high-risk, high-volume and/or problem-prone areas are monitored.

IV. Quality philosophy and framework
1. Leadership's PI structure and responsibilities
   A. Overview of the hospital's PI structure, accompanied by an organizational chart
   B. Board of directors' responsibilities
   C. Medical staff's responsibilities
   D. Hospital administration's responsibilities

   Briefly describe each entity or committee's purpose, including what types of data it will review and what authority and responsibility it has, including communication with constituencies.

2. Performance improvement model
   Describe your hospital's PI model.

3. Information and analysis
   Describe your information resources for PI.

4. Human resource development and management
   Describe your training resources and how PI is integrated with management and performance reviews.

5. Patient and customer focus and satisfaction
   Link these to performance measures.

6. Outcomes and results
   Describe which indicators are monitored by the quality governing committee and the board; describe the annual self-assessment process.

APPENDICES

I. Quality goals for the current year

II. Sections and organizational units
   A. Medical staff departments/sections
   B. Hospital departments/units
      List in detail the units included in the scope of the PI program.

III. Confidentiality guidelines
Restate the hospital's confidentiality policy here briefly.

IV. Highlights of changes from the prior year's plan

This preamble should be revisited annually through the self-assessment process and the annual management and board review of the PI plan, but as it is linked to the overall mission of the hospital, it will not be subject to frequent change.

Scope of the performance improvement program

Be sure to describe your scope of services, such as inpatient, outpatient, ambulatory surgery, adult, pediatric, emergency department, home health, and clinics or owned physician practices. This statement should match both the scope documents you submit to JCAHO with your survey application every 3 years and any other hospital documents describing your scope of services.

Organization

Somewhere in your PI plan, you should describe how the hospital will bring people and resources together to achieve its PI goals. Usually, this section of the PI plan briefly reviews the PI responsibilities of the governing body and all levels of hospital leaders, including managers, clinical chairs, and chiefs. You may want to include an organization chart outlining the board's overall responsibility and how other committees report to them.

Depending on the needs of the audience, you may want to describe each leadership group's role in PI and each quality committee's charter as well, so that the plan is a concise summary of the entire organization's resources for PI. Generally, this type of information is found in medical staff and governing board bylaws as well as in quality committee charters.

This section of the PI plan should also outline which resources have been committed by the organization to support PI, such as the quality support department and medical records department, who can train staff and support your statistical or information systems and benchmarking efforts. You do not need to supply much detail, but a quick overview of major resources will help you respond to a number of surveyor inquiries efficiently.

Approach to selecting improvement priorities

Somewhere in your PI plan, you should describe the methodology used by management and medical staff leadership to identify annual improvement priorities. You may describe this approach in a general statement that refers the reader back to the JCAHO's own priority-setting criteria, or you may choose to define a more complex and specific process the hospital might use, such as multivoting or a point-scoring system. For instance, this section might read, "The quality oversight committee will identify annual hospital-wide PI priorities through consensus, based on a review of the annual self-assessment and other pertinent measures and inputs such as community needs. The priorities may be adjusted throughout the year as new findings and measures become available."

The goal is to succinctly describe how the hospital ensures that it assesses important populations and processes to look for PI opportunities. It is sufficient to simply state that you will ensure that they receive attention; you do not need to go into the mechanics of the process here. However, it may be helpful for you to include more specifics in this portion of the plan, depending on how you will use the plan to educate your internal audiences. For instance, you may describe some simple and clear "rules" for how managers should propose a project for a PI team, such as "The PI oversight committee will receive proposals each quarter and will charter PI teams according to the format in appendix 1." You do not need to be this specific in the PI plan, however.

Chapter 8

NOTE: When JCAHO surveyors interview the PI oversight committee, or whatever structure governs the PI process in the hospital (see Chapter 3 for more information) they will ask how the hospital sets its priorities. These surveyors want to see that the hospital has a thoughtful and comprehensive priority-setting process in place. Of course, if your priority-setting system is documented in the PI plan, then the committee's discussion should reflect that methodology. If it is not documented in the plan, you should demonstrate that there is a process and that it is consistently used.

Information flow
You also should define who will receive reports on the progress of PI teams. At a minimum, you should define the responsibilities of each group that will review this information. This may be incorporated most efficiently into each committee description, such as, "The PI oversight committee will meet monthly. Every PI team and hospital department will submit measures quarterly on a rotating schedule so that the oversight committee is able to monitor performance continuously."

Confidentiality provisions
Be sure to restate or refer to the hospital's overall confidentiality policy somewhere in the plan. In this statement, you should make special reference to unique confidentiality requirements and describe any provisions for the confidentiality of quality and PI data (e.g., your state may extend special protection to quality-related processes and information).

Approach to the annual self-assessment or evaluation of the performance improvement program
Each year, the hospital's PI program should be thoroughly assessed by the quality oversight committee, and that self-assessment should be reviewed and approved by the board of directors. This step fulfills both the letter and the spirit of a number of JCAHO requirements in PI and leadership.

The PI plan merely needs to affirm that this assessment will be performed and to outline how the information will flow to the appropriate parties. For example, you might state that "The PI oversight committee will receive a self-assessment of each team's and department's PI activities each year. This will be forwarded to the quality committee of the board of directors for approval and the results will be used to establish next year's PI plan." (See Chapter 11 for more information on assessment.)

Detailed annual goals
The PI plan doesn't have to list 100% of each year's specific PI goals for the hospital. The logistics of collecting and publishing all goals from throughout the hospital would be overwhelming, and it would be impractical to revise and reapprove the plan each time any of the individual goals changed. However, it is wise to include a brief appendix to the plan containing the highest-priority multidisciplinary and interdepartmental goals that will require hospital-wide focus. Following this format will ensure that the PI plan communicates the year's priorities unmistakably and that the PI plan serves as a reference document all year long.

Most hospitals have a few major improvement goals that are likely to demand attention from the entire hospital, such as

- Improving overall patient satisfaction
- Improving physician satisfaction with laboratory, radiology, and other ancillary reporting of test results

- Improving nosocomial infection rates
- Reducing lengths of stay while maintaining quality outcomes in the top 10 DRGs

In some cases, the plan may include goals that are not hospital-wide but that are a focus for the entire hospital. For example, if the hospital has recently started a new clinical program, it may be advisable for the whole organization to recognize that there is a hospital-wide goal to "improve efficiency and quality outcomes of the new cardiac surgery program." Every area, from information systems to transportation, marketing, and admitting, can contribute to this quality goal.

NOTE: Some hospitals supply a copy of their PI plans to managed care firms wishing to determine whether the hospital has a comprehensive PI program. It is advisable to supply the plan without details on the current year's goals; an "appendix" structure for the goals allows you to simply omit that section when sharing the plan.

Securing approval of the performance improvement plan

Once you've finished drafting the PI plan, it should be reviewed by several members of its intended audience, such as clinical managers and directors, to ensure that it is both readable and usable. It should then be formally reviewed and approved by the hospital's PI oversight committee. As these individuals look it over, they should pay special attention to the listed annual goals and any major changes that have been made to the hospital's PI program (e.g., changing committee functions).

Once the oversight committee's approval has been secured, you should then bring the PI plan to the board of directors for approval. An effective method is to use one meeting each year to present the prior year's self-assessment and this year's new PI plan all at once. This demonstrates the connection between the two and shows the continuous improvement philosophy in action.

Remember, the board members will be asked by JCAHO surveyors to discuss how each year's plan is established, how they know it is responsive to the community you seek to serve, and how they feel comfortable that it encompasses all major populations in the hospital. Be sure to offer them all of this information when you present them with the PI plan.

Distributing the performance improvement plan

When the PI plan is finalized, be sure to share it with all executives, managers, and medical leaders in the hospital. This will help inform them of some of their most important PI priorities for the coming year.

Notes

Chapter 9

Designing New Processes and Programs (PI.2)

The goal is simple. To be in compliance with the *Comprehensive Accreditation Manual for Hospitals (CAMH)* standard PI.2, hospital managers and leaders, including PI oversight committees, must consider the hospital's performance goals as they establish new or significantly change any services, programs, product lines, buildings, or processes.

What this means is that before a new process is designed, leaders should reflect on the hospital's mission, vision, PI plan, patient and staff expectations, and external information about processes at other hospitals, and incorporate these issues into the process's design. In addition, revisions to standard PI.2 require hospitals to ensure that their process follows "sound business practices," and hospitals should consider how the program or service will perform compared to its baseline, or starting level.

Read through this chapter for advice on how to ensure that your hospital's processes are all designed or redesigned in accordance with standard PI.2.

Why is it important to design new processes in accordance with performance improvement principles?

If there is a single overriding insight in the total quality management literature of the past 50 years, it is this: *Quality is designed into a process.* Quality is not achieved by inspecting the product of a haphazard process and critiquing it; a truly quality process is designed with careful attention to the desired result from the beginning.

It is absolutely true that healthcare processes are unique to each patient. It is true that we have processes of mind-boggling complexity and innumerable variables. And it is true that we cannot give up post-hoc quality analyses, such as the study of "defects" (e.g., complications, mortality rates, undesirable waiting times, and complaints)—although neither the Joint Commission on Accreditation of Healthcare Organizations (JCAHO) nor leading quality thinkers would prescribe this. However, we cannot solely study problems to improve quality. To develop reliable, consistent processes, we must fully understand these systems and be sufficiently committed to high-quality outcomes from the start.

Healthcare is not a "production function" like a factory, and therefore our processes have to be designed for tremendous flexibility. Each process must have room for timely professional

Chapter 9

judgment and patient participation in care and treatment decisions. Today's clinical pathways, clinical algorithms, and treatment guidelines are evidence that systematic PI thinking can result in the development of processes that successfully marry flexibility and planning.

Incorporating JCAHO design requirements into your business planning and performance improvement frameworks

One of the most effective ways of ensuring that your hospital meets the requirements listed in JCAHO's standard PI.2 is to incorporate the standard's provisions into the hospital's business planning and PI frameworks.

If the hospital has a formal planning methodology, perhaps for all projects exceeding a given investment threshold, basic process and quality criteria can be readily incorporated into that framework. This will immediately address process design compliance for such areas as acquisition and implementation of new imaging technology or the construction of new patient care areas.

For example, a business planning framework for laparoscopy should address such basic quality issues as these:

- Why is the procedure needed in our community?
- What are all financial considerations (e.g., the cost of acquiring the equipment)?
- What are all staffing considerations (e.g., competency of supporting personnel as well as credentials of the physicians performing the procedure)?
- What are all environmental and process considerations (e.g., sterilization procedures, preventive maintenance)?
- What are all safety and performance measures (e.g., complications, conversions to open cases)?

All new processes should also be designed in accordance with the hospital's chosen PI model, or framework. Whether the hospital uses an established PI model (e.g., Deming's "plan, do, check, act") or has developed its own, the PI plan and other supporting materials, such as training manuals, will describe how this framework should be used to create or redesign processes. Before you begin to design a new process, take a brief look through these documents to ensure that you fully understand your PI model's requirements.

Documenting the design of a process

Documents such as a business plan, minutes, and supporting data accumulated by a development team or, even better, presentation materials or storyboards from such teams, or both, and press releases, articles, and advertisements in employee or external publications, or all three, can all demonstrate compliance with the PI.2 standards to surveyors.

For purposes of the triennial JCAHO survey, you have to pull together these documents for only a few programs, not every single one in the hospital. You simply need to show that the hospital considers performance when it designs a new process and follows through when the process is implemented.

Chapter 10

Performance Measurement: The Key to Your Performance Improvement Program's Success (PI.3)

For many hospitals, performance measurement can be confusing and overwhelming. In part, this is because there's plenty of information available to explain performance improvement (PI) theories but very little helpful "how-to" advice on how to implement them. This lack of practical information and guidance has caused innumerable problems for hospitals. For example, many hospitals

- Measure too much or don't measure enough
- Lack a clear sense of what data they should be gathering on a consistent basis
- Fail to measure Joint Commission on the Accreditation of Healthcare Organizations (JCAHO)–required elements
- Collect data that serve no useful purpose, thereby wasting energy and inviting surveyor challenges
- Overlook opportunities to improve staff satisfaction, efficiency, and effectiveness (issues that must be addressed to meet JCAHO standards)

Yet, in spite of these problems, it is possible to develop a useful set of measures for your hospital. Although it's true that every hospital has different priorities, and it's impossible to develop one perfect set of measures that will meet every organization's needs, each hospital must conduct a number of measurements required by the Joint Commission. Read through this chapter to learn just how to select a set of measures that will meet JCAHO standards and help you to develop an effective PI program for your hospital.

Why measure at all?

Measurement is an important part of PI simply because *without measurement you cannot show improvement!* The entire idea of performance or outcomes depends on some type of evaluation or measurement of a process. The measurement may be subjective, impressionistic, objective, or invalid—but some type of measurement must be conducted before you can determine what problems should be addressed. After all, how do we know that something is better (or not better!) unless we have measured it?

These very simple concepts can be easily forgotten in an environment that is focused too heavily on JCAHO compliance. For example, many hospitals develop PI measures just for the sake of having measures to show to surveyors, and they don't take the time to ensure that their measures are thoughtful, well constructed, and will help achieve the hospital's annual goals.

To avoid this problem, you should remember that measurement is the process of collecting data to be used to assess performance and does not exist as an independent activity. All measurements must be driven by your intended purpose. For example, it may be convenient to collect diagnosis data on a patient's admission to the hospital, and this would be useful if you were studying the effectiveness of your bed-assignment system to match patients' diagnoses with units devoted to certain clinical problems. However, data on diagnosis at admission will not be useful if you want to assess clinical outcomes 6 weeks after discharge; for this purpose, you would most likely need to know the diagnosis at discharge.

Meeting JCAHO standards

The Joint Commission no longer requires hospitals to implement measurements continuously within every one of the 11 functions listed in its *Comprehensive Accreditation Manual for Hospitals* (*CAMH*) (Patient's Rights and Organizational Ethics, Assessment of Patients, Performance Improvement, etc.). Now their requirements focus instead on aspects of patient care, and most of them cross function lines. This book provides checklists to help you match your PI projects with JCAHO requirements.

For full JCAHO compliance, it is essential that you evaluate all of the performance measures stipulated. JCAHO does not demand that you use any particular improvement model, computer system, team approach, or governing process. With the exception of core performance measures (in process of implementation during 2000–2002), JCAHO does not tell you exactly what to measure, how to conduct the measurement itself, or how often to examine the results.

What is required is that you evaluate the JCAHO's nine "dimensions" of performance as you conduct performance measures:

- Efficacy—the ability of the process to improve patient care
- Appropriateness—choosing the right measure to use in improving particular patients' care
- Availability—the degree to which the process is available to those who need it when and where they need it
- Timeliness—provision of service at the right time
- Effectiveness—how well the process works to improve patient care
- Continuity—how well the process works to assure patient care throughout the course of treatment
- Safety—how well the process helps maintain a safe environment for patient care
- Efficiency—how well the appropriate practice is undertaken in a timely fashion
- Respect/dignity—how well the process preserves the respect and dignity to which all patients and staff are entitled

We can consider these dimensions as responses to two questions:

- *Did we do the right thing?*
- *Did we do it well?*

In the course of a JCAHO survey, you will probably need to show which dimensions of performance apply to any given project. You are not required to measure all nine dimensions of performance for every measure you take. When JCAHO surveyors interview a PI team, the group should be able to discuss all of the dimensions of performance that mattered in the improvement. Review each PI measure with your team so that team members are familiar with all of the dimensions of performance that pertain. Figure 10.1 provides a checklist of JCAHO-defined dimensions of performance and areas of patient care you can use to describe a particular PI project.

The hospital should assess all nine dimensions of performance over the course of 1 year. If you find in your review that any of these dimensions is missing, consider refocusing the quality program in your hospital. For example, if no one is evaluating safety or respect and dignity, then this is a gap that deserves attention. You can use Figure 10.2 to discover which JCAHO requirements your PI projects meet. You must have at least one project in place in each of the required measurement areas (operative and invasive procedures, blood administration, etc.), and measure dimensions of performance with one project or other.

Measuring other JCAHO-required elements

As noted previously, the JCAHO requires you to conduct performance measurements throughout the hospital and to evaluate the pertinent dimensions of performance for each measurement you take. In addition to these general requirements, the JCAHO has developed a list of 11 specific areas in which hospitals must implement performance measurement:

- Operative and invasive procedures
- Patient treatment: blood administration (ordering, distributing, administering, monitoring)
- Patient treatment: medication administration (ordering, dispensing, administering, monitoring)
- Patient treatment: restraint and seclusion
- Patient/customer satisfaction and perception of care and service
- High-risk, high-volume, and problem-prone processes
- Newly designed or redesigned processes
- Requirements from other *CAMH* chapters
- Resuscitation outcomes
- Sentinel events
- Adverse events

Many hospitals have trouble combining these required measurement areas with their own improvement goals, and they wind up adding measures that feel meaningless in an attempt to satisfy the JCAHO. This is largely because the JCAHO's requirements are so ambiguous; the standards do not explain what you should measure in each key area. For example, the JCAHO leaves it up to you to decide how to measure blood administration performance in your hospital. Should you measure documentation accuracy? Incident reports? Technical competence? The standards don't lead us to select one set of measures over another, because they recognize that

Chapter 10

FIGURE 10.1

How a performance improvement project meets JCAHO requirements

Name of PI project
_____
_____

Check all that apply.

Dimensions of performance
- ❏ Efficacy
- ❏ Appropriateness
- ❏ Availability
- ❏ Timeliness
- ❏ Effectiveness
- ❏ Continuity
- ❏ Safety
- ❏ Efficiency
- ❏ Respect and dignity

Areas of patient care

- ❏ **Patient rights and organization ethics (RI)**
- ❏ Patient satisfaction
- ❏ Advance directives, informed consent
- ❏ **Assessment of patients (PE)**
- ❏ Especially related to pain[1]
- ❏ **Care of patients (TX)**
- ❏ Operative and invasive procedures
- ❏ • Patient selection
- ❏ • Patient preparation
- ❏ • Patient education
- ❏ • Performance of procedure
- ❏ • Post-procedure monitoring
- ❏ Blood administration
- ❏ • Ordering
- ❏ • Distributing
- ❏ • Administering
- ❏ • Monitoring
- ❏ Medication administration
- ❏ • Ordering
- ❏ • Distributing
- ❏ • Administering
- ❏ • Monitoring
- ❏ Restraints and seclusion
- ❏ • Measures for behavioral health
- ❏ • Measures for medical/surgical patients

- ❏ **Patient and family education (PF)**
- ❏ Language/cultural competence
- ❏ Assessment
- ❏ Documentation
- ❏ Pain management[1]
- ❏ **Continuum of care (CC)**
   See Utilization Review under PI
- ❏ **Improving organizational performance (PI)**
- ❏ High-risk activities
- ❏ High-volume activities
- ❏ Problem-prone activities
- ❏ Newly designed/redesigned processes
- ❏ Resuscitation outcomes
- ❏ Sentinel events
- ❏ Adverse events/Risk management
- ❏ ORYX measures for our hospital
- ❏ Pain management[1]
- ❏ Clinical guideline use and outcomes[1]
- ❏ Utilization management[2]
- ❏ Staff views of performance[2]
- ❏ Autopsy results[2]
- ❏ Quality control, where appropriate
- ❏ **Leadership (LD)**
- ❏ **Management of the environment of care (CC)**
- ❏ **Management of human resources (HR)**
- ❏ **Management of information (IM)**
- ❏ **Surveillance, prevention, and control of infection (IC)**

[1] New standard for focus.
[2] Area to consider (not required).

FIGURE 10.2

Mapping performance improvement measurements to JCAHO requirements

By mapping some of your hospital's PI projects to the JCAHO's required areas and dimensions of measurement, you'll be able to demonstrate that the hospital measures its performance in each of the areas of patient care required by the Joint Commission for performance measurement activity.

This form will help you prepare for your JCAHO accreditation survey. It will not list all the PI activities you have in place. Its purpose is to show that you meet the requirements for improvement in all critical aspects of patient care (as defined by the Joint Commission) and that your projects measure all of the JCAHO-defined "dimensions" of performance in one way or another.

Checkpoints:

- Are all dimensions measured somewhere?
- Are all required functions measured with at least some relevant dimensions?
- Did we use a single measurement to meet multiple requirements wherever possible and appropriate, to focus our energy on really achieving improvement rather than excess measures?
- Can we demonstrate that we have considered the other (nonrequired) functions for possible measurement?

Directions: For each JCAHO-required performance area, list a PI project you have in place. Then check the dimension of patient care this project measures.

JCAHO-required performance measurement area	Your hospital's PI projects	JCAHO-defined dimensions of patient care								
		Efficacy	Appropriateness	Availability	Timeliness	Effectiveness	Continuity	Safety	Efficiency	Respect/dignity
Operative and invasive procedures[1] • Patient selection • Patient preparation • Patient education • Performance of procedure • Post-procedure monitoring										
Blood administration[1] • Ordering • Distributing • Administering • Monitoring										

FIGURE 10.2 *(cont'd)*

JCAHO-required performance measurement area	Your hospital's PI projects	JCAHO-defined dimensions of patient care								
		Efficacy	Appropriateness	Availability	Timeliness	Effectiveness	Continuity	Safety	Efficiency	Respect/dignity
Medication administration[1] • Ordering • Distributing • Administering • Monitoring										
Restraints and seclusion (measures for behavioral health): aggregate data by • Unit • Shift • Purpose • Type of staff • Multiple episodes per patient										
Restraints and seclusion (measures for medical/surgical patients)										
No specific requirements for aggregating data; you select appropriate measures										
Patient satisfaction										
High-risk activities										
High-volume activities										
Problem-prone activities										
Newly designed/redesigned processes										
Requirements from other *CAMH* chapters[2] • Patient rights, advance directives, consent										

FIGURE 10.2 (cont'd)

• Patient and family education • Patient assessment (pain management; documentation) • Medical records documentation (information management) • Competence • Infection control • Environment of care • Leadership, PI, governance, medical staff, etc.								
Resuscitation outcomes								
Sentinel events								
Adverse events/risk management								
Selected ORYX/core measures (six ORYX measures implemented by 12/31/99)								
Pain management[3]								
Clinical guideline use and outcomes[3]								
Utilization management[4]								
Staff views of performance[4]								
Autopsy results[4]								
Quality control, where appropriate[4]								

[1]Must show measurement and assessment in each of these required elements and improvement as appropriate; you may address all of the elements in a single PI initiative or in separate ones.
[2]Measurement and assessment must be in place for each function; a single PI initiative may address several different areas at once.
[3]New standards for focus.
[4]Areas to consider (not required).

each hospital is its own best judge of where measurement is needed. But this lack of specificity can lead to confusion and concern about meeting accreditation requirements.

Therefore, you should concentrate on using the required measurement categories as a structure, a framework, within which you will choose measures to help you meet your hospital's own improvement priorities. For example, you are required to measure blood ordering, preparation, administration, and monitoring of patient response. If you know that your documentation on blood use is flawless, don't waste your time measuring its quality. Focus your efforts instead on measuring areas about which you're not as confident, such as perhaps nursing technical competence (maybe you can simultaneously improve your compliance with the Human Resources standards for staff competence!) or the quality and thoroughness of incident reports related to transfusion reactions. As one surveyor advised, "Don't keep measuring what you know is working fine; focus on areas where you think you can make improvements."

One word of caution: You must be able to demonstrate that you conduct measures in each of these 11 required areas. In earlier years, surveyors were more or less content to see that hospitals conducted a few measurements in some of the required areas, but as surveyors become more and more comfortable with the contemporary approach to PI, they will be tougher on this standard. They will expect hospitals to not only conduct measurements in all the required areas but also to be more creative in their PI activities and take on real challenges in the PI program.

Read through the following information to better understand how to approach each measurement and what pitfalls you should avoid. In addition, we've listed sample measurements in some of the more complex sections to help you get started. As you read, use the matrix in Figure 10.2 to check off the required areas in which you know you have measures in place. You should find that you are readily able to think of projects that include measurement and improvement in all required categories. Remember that it is acceptable for one project to satisfy measurement requirements in more than one category.

Operative and invasive procedures

The JCAHO requires hospitals to measure how well

- Patients are selected and prepared for operative and invasive procedures
- Patients are educated about the procedure
- All operative and invasive procedures are performed
- Patients are cared for post-procedure

The Joint Commission intends that this performance review will present a good assessment of the entire process surrounding invasive procedures.

Remember, the JCAHO doesn't require you to conduct "operative and invasive procedure" reviews on all high-volume procedures, but surveyors will want to see that you review a credible group of operative procedures. This demonstrates to the surveyors that selection of patients, preparation of patients, performance of the procedure, and post-procedure care and patient education are effectively performed in the hospital.

The annual PI plan (hospital-wide and departmental plans, or both) should note which procedures will be measured and which measures will be conducted for each procedure. Then, staff from nursing and medical departments, operating rooms, and procedural areas can conduct these measurements.

There may be areas in which you do not think that all components of a procedure need to be measured and assessed. For example, perhaps staff wants to focus only on how a certain procedure is performed and aren't concerned about the quality of pre- or post-procedure care. That is not a problem. The JCAHO doesn't require you to measure all five of the listed issues for each and every operative and invasive procedure, though this is usually the most convenient way to minimize the number of patient records that need to be reviewed and assessed. If the quality department agrees, staff can measure only the quality of patient education for one procedure, the quality of pre-procedure care for another, and so on.

Most likely, a number of your hospital's operative and invasive procedures will be classified as high-risk, high-volume, and/or problem-prone. These procedures can be targeted for measurement under the high-risk requirement. If this is the case, indicators for these already highlighted procedures can merely be refined. For instance, if the gastrointestinal laboratory identifies colonoscopy as a high-volume, high-risk, and/or problem-prone process, you should ensure that you measure selection of patients, preparation of patients, performance of the procedure, post-procedure care, and patient education to meet JCAHO requirements.

Patient treatment: blood administration (ordering, distributing, administering, monitoring)

You must study how well blood is ordered, distributed, administered, and monitored in your hospital on a regular basis.

With the current national focus on medical errors, this is a good place to consider studying the literature and emerging clinical practice guidelines. Also, consider integrating sentinel event and risk management monitoring to incorporate several required measurements in one initiative.

As with medication use, this requirement affects the practices of a number of departments, such as the medical staff, nursing, and the blood bank, and would therefore probably be best monitored through an interdisciplinary group or committee. Often the hospital's blood or transfusion committee monitors these measures, but if that is not practical for your organization, the quality or nursing department or possibly the blood bank may collect the gathered measurement data and disseminate it to all relevant disciplines.

No matter who collects this measurement data, indicators should be set up and reviewed annually. For example, your hospital might decide to measure how well it

- Obtains consent to use blood
- Secures signed physician orders that specify all pertinent information (e.g., rate of administration)
- Delivers blood in a timely manner
- Stores blood before it is administered
- Manages transfusion reactions

Again, if there is a standing blood use committee, it should be in charge of measuring this data. Remember, if you don't have a standing interdisciplinary group, it may be difficult to attain shared focus on the issues.

Patient treatment: medication administration (ordering, dispensing, administering, monitoring)

As with blood administration (see previous section), medication administration is one of the primary focus areas for national concern regarding medical errors and reduction of patient mortality and morbidity associated with errors. You should pay close attention to emerging clinical practice guidelines in this area, and this is an ideal place to integrate other required measurements, such as sentinel event monitoring, perhaps invasive procedure review, nursing practice and documentation reviews, etc. A significant area such as this one can effectively integrate many areas of required measurement, making your work more efficient and improving patient care in a more immediate and integrated fashion.

The Joint Commission requires you to measure how well medication is ordered, dispensed, administered, and monitored in your hospital. You should focus your attention both on medications that are high-volume, high-risk, and problem-prone, or all three, and on a sampling of other medications whose use you think could be improved. All four of the JCAHO's medication use activities (e.g., ordering, distributing, administering, and monitoring) must be evaluated periodically.

Generally, these measures reflect activities of several disciplines, such as the medical, nursing, and pharmacy staffs, and are usually conducted or overseen by the hospital's pharmacy and therapeutics committee. Sample indicators may include signed physician orders; patient consent for drugs identified by the committee as high-risk; appropriate use of experimental drugs; dispensing and labeling accuracy; pharmacist counseling; timely and accurate administration; or the timely monitoring after medications are administered, including documentation of adverse reactions.

Patient treatment: restraint and seclusion

Restraint and seclusion have always been modes of treatment that we are reluctant to use, because they clearly interfere with a patient's right to freedom of movement. These are selected for use only when essential for a patient's own well-being and the protection of other patients and staff. The Joint Commission has for many years enforced fairly stringent standards for measurement and trending of data involving any problems in restraints, including apparent excessive use, negative outcomes, etc. However, with the escalation of concerns about restraint use to the federal level and the publication of formal and strict guidelines in the *Medicare Conditions of Participation* in August 1999, the JCAHO is responding with its own heightened focus.

You must be aware of the federal rules (see Bibliography) and continue to monitor JCAHO developments. JCAHO standards are inconsistent with federal rules, and as always the stricter standards apply. The variances between the two are not great, but the Joint Commission is in the process of updating its standards to meet and perhaps exceed the federal ones.

If you continue to perform all of the measurements outlined in the JCAHO standards as currently written and are careful to monitor the Health Care Financing Administration (HCFA) rules related to physician evaluation and restraint orders, you should be able to meet both sets of standards and continue to assure good patient care.

You can expect surveyors to be well-educated in the HCFA standards when they visit your facility and ask you how you are ensuring that you do meet the federal requirements as well as the JCAHO ones.

The JCAHO continues to have two sets of required measures for restraint and seclusion use. As always with mandated measures, your documentation must demonstrate that there was actual review and assessment of these aggregated data. If you decided not to intervene to improve your restraint process, you should be able to show why you concluded that performance was acceptable.

For behavioral health patients

(Note that the use of restraints or seclusion for behavioral health patients standard applies to patients who are receiving services in a psychiatric service. It does not apply to use of restraints, even for behavior control or psychiatric problems, if the patient is in a general acute medical-surgical unit. This is different from the approach of HCFA's new standards issued in August 1999, in which the purpose of the restraint determines whether medical-surgical or psychiatric standards apply.)

To meet JCAHO requirements, measurement must include 100% review of all charts and data collected and aggregated for all units, all shifts, all purposes, multiple episodes of use, and frequency of use by type of staff.

For medical-surgical patients

Measurement of restraint or seclusion use for medical-surgical patients is targeted to understanding the reasons for restraint use and need not cover 100% of episodes of use, nor need it cover predefined elements. The JCAHO recommends the development of a targeted measurement program based on an initial baseline assessment, which all hospitals should have in place from earlier years when 100% measurement was required for all restraint episodes. Using this baseline, or a new one, you should show in your documentation how you've decided what data to continue to collect. It is evident that some type of measurement, even if based on random sampling, certain populations or processes, or other methods, must continue; and the goal of your program must clearly be to reduce the use of restraints.

Patient satisfaction

The JCAHO remains somewhat vague about the patient satisfaction standard. The needs and expectations of patients and others about performance can be measured in a number of ways.

The vast majority of hospitals today use some form of patient satisfaction survey (e.g., paper, telephone, electronic, or in-person surveys) to assess whether needs and expectations were met. No requirement in the standard states that surveying per se should be performed, nor that 100% of patients should be assessed, nor that benchmarking should be conducted to compare the hospital's results to those of others—although this is a good idea, and if it were done, it would meet other standards for comparative data analysis in both the PI and information management chapters.

High-risk, high-volume, and problem-prone processes

The JCAHO requires hospitals to measure all of their high-risk, high-volume, and problem-prone processes. But before a hospital can put any such measurements in place, it must determine which of its processes fall into this category. The objective is to take inventory of all key processes and implement measurements in each high-priority area.

The best way to develop this inventory is to encourage both the hospital's PI oversight committee and each department manager to brainstorm and determine which processes are high-risk, high-volume, and problem-prone. For example, the hospital's PI oversight committee could brainstorm to develop a comprehensive list of all of the "high-risk, high-volume, and problem-prone" processes in the entire hospital. In addition, every manager in the hospital could develop his or her own list of which key processes in his or her area should be monitored.

Ideally, every hospital department should conduct such a brief planning exercise each year to establish how it will define, measure, and improve performance in all high-risk, high-volume, and problem-prone processes. (See Chapters 6 and 7 for more information on the mechanics of this process.)

Newly designed or redesigned processes

As noted in Chapter 9, planning for new programs and services or for major changes in services should always be done with some basic attention to how you want the program to perform. For instance, a new skilled nursing facility may be designed for timely admission, patient dignity, and cost-effectiveness (thereby addressing the functions of patient assessment and continuum of care and the dimensions of performance of timeliness, appropriateness, and continuity of care).

Anyone who will be designing a new process or implementing a change to a process should be taught how to design measures that will effectively monitor the improved process to confirm that it remains improved. For example, if the pharmacy expands its hours into the evening, there may automatically be a cost/benefit analysis that compares the new revenues to the cost of staff time and other expenses. There could also be measures of patient satisfaction, more timely discharges, maybe even staff satisfaction. Ideally, the hospital's business planning framework or hospital planning process (see Chapter 9) will explicitly address measures of quality and performance up front as new systems, programs, and processes are designed.

Sentinel events and adverse events

The JCAHO enacted sentinel event standards for 1999. In PI.4.3, the JCAHO requires you to "intensively analyze" sentinel events and other "undesirable patterns or trends in performance." The JCAHO defines a *sentinel event* as "an unexpected occurrence involving death or serious physical or psychological injury, or the risk thereof."

You also have a wider field of data, including events that do not reach the level of a JCAHO-defined "sentinel" event but have the potential of tragic consequences ("close call" or "near miss" events). In the risk management program, you can trend and improve processes that may be generating preventable adverse events. Formerly, JCAHO standards required measurement in risk management; this is now technically optional. Because adverse event monitoring is required, the effect is the same. You will certainly need to continue tracking and trending patterns in risk management data to meet the standard on addressing adverse events.

In educating your hospital community, you want to emphasize that you are interested in reducing all preventable adverse events, and that a subset of these events may reach the threshold of a JCAHO-defined "sentinel event." It is important that we keep focused on the widest possible field of errors and potential errors to reduce them. If staff believe that they only need to focus on avoiding "sentinel" events, they will have missed the entire principle of risk management, prevention of "adverse events," and the national focus on reducing medical error overall.

PI.4.4 requires hospitals to take action to "reduce the risk of sentinel events." To comply with this standard, your hospital should use the information from data analyses and root-cause analyses to improve performance and reduce the risk of sentinel events. Also, your hospital must have a system in place to perform self-assessments when leaders become aware of sentinel events at other hospitals. This includes events described in the JCAHO's ongoing series of sentinel event bulletins, *Sentinel Event Alert*.

The Intent statement for standard PI.3.1.1 makes it clear that you must pay attention to sentinel and adverse events at other organizations. This includes patterns of events, such as confusion between two similarly named drugs, which might be identified by other facilities or the Joint Commission. Your quality committee should address these issues as they appear and should discuss initiating such self-assessments. Examine both single sentinel events and patterns of events to determine whether your facility should take preventive measures, and remember to fully document this discussion.

The JCAHO wants its reporting system and sentinel events database to trigger this kind of interhospital comparison and proactive assessment. Based on information already collected, the JCAHO's *Sentinel Event Alerts* identify event risks and offer prevention advice. At the very minimum, quality and risk managers should monitor these *Alerts* and keep their quality oversight committees informed of important industry trends. (Your hospital is certainly already receiving the Joint Commission's *Alerts*; an archive of past *Alerts* is available at www.jcaho.org/edu_pub/sealert/se_alert.html.)

Figure 10.3 contains some core elements of the JCAHO's sentinel event policy. To help create your own sentinel events policy (and to provide examples of compliance), use Appendix 3. For more information, see the Joint Commission's Web page offering links to its information about sentinel and adverse events: www.jcaho.org/sentinel/sentevnt_main.html. Their Sentinel Event Hotline telephone number is 630/792-3700.

In LD.4.3.1, the JCAHO requires leaders to define and implement the processes for identifying and managing sentinel events. According to the JCAHO, hospital leaders are responsible for establishing a culture that is conducive to the identification, reporting, analysis, and prevention of sentinel events, and for ensuring the consistent and effective implementation of a mechanism to accomplish these activities. This mechanism should include the completion of a root-cause analysis—an in-depth investigation to determine why a sentinel event occurred.

Adverse events

The Assessment standard PI.4.3 highlights the types of events (beyond sentinel events) that must trigger intensive assessment:

- Performance is significantly worse than expected
- Performance is significantly worse than other organizations
- Performance is significantly worse than recognized standards
- Confirmed transfusion reactions
- Significant adverse drug reactions
- Significant medication errors (the standard offers a specific definition of these last two)
- Major discrepancies between preoperative and postoperative diagnoses
- Significant adverse events associated with anesthesia use

FIGURE 10.3

Core elements of the JCAHO's sentinel event policy

A definition of a sentinel event approved by leaders and communicated throughout the hospital

Your hospital must be able to identify—and describe the methods used to identify—potential sentinel events as the JCAHO defines them. Your hospital must also be able to investigate them systematically and in a timely manner. Your risk management or quality department should probably be responsible for these activities—with significant input from legal counsel.

Established channels for reporting sentinel events within the hospital and to regulatory and accrediting bodies

Your hospital must have a process in place to determine how to ensure compliance with the JCAHO policy, including possible voluntary self-reporting. In other words, your hospital's leaders should be able to explain who will decide if and when to make a voluntary report of a confirmed sentinel event at your hospital. Not only does the JCAHO require organizations to create such a process under LD.4.3.1, but also it's just common sense for your hospital's leaders to know in advance how they will handle a sentinel event if it ever occurs.

A process for conducting a thorough root-cause analysis that focuses on process and systems factors, with an associated risk reduction plan

Your hospital must prepare a root-cause analysis of each sentinel event in a timely manner. Your hospital should be able to identify a specific person or department as driving the root-cause analysis process.

An action plan that includes measuring the effectiveness of process and system improvements to reduce risk

Your hospital must have a process in place to identify and implement systems changes and other improvement initiatives to deal with the root cause(s) identified during analyses. You should be able to identify a specific group or department—such as the quality committee or the governing board—that is charged with reviewing root-cause analyses and authorizing improvement plans.

To assess these, obviously you must have data collection methods in place to identify them and trigger such an assessment.

Benchmarking and ORYX/core measure requirements: other considerations in designing and selecting measures

The hospital should use comparative measures from leading hospitals to gather data on key processes. For example, your organization might choose to select comparative measures from the JCAHO's national database of leading comparative measures or the federal Agency for Health Care Policy Research's database, Conquest, which is available free on the Internet. By using these measures to compare your practices to those of other organizations, you can determine whether your hospital is in line with industry standards.

To make valid comparisons, you will need to design measurements in the same manner as your selected benchmarks. For example, if you are going to compare your hospital's performance to that of another hospital, you must conduct your measure exactly as the comparison hospital did. If that hospital collected data "from the minute the physician order to admit has been signed until the patient is physically in the new bed," you must collect data using those parameters as well. This is the only way you can ensure that your comparisons are accurate and useful. See Chapter 6 for more details on designing measurements.

The JCAHO's ORYX program, implemented in 1997, added another twist to its benchmarking requirements. Each hospital selected clinical performance measures from a list of JCAHO-approved performance measurement systems that reflected the care provided to its patients in areas of clinical importance. Hospitals collected these measures, sent their results to the approved system, and authorized that system to give the hospital's outcomes data to the JCAHO quarterly.

These ORYX requirements placed new and challenging demands on hospitals, but they are already being superseded by the JCAHO's emerging new program for a smaller, more focused, and much more demanding set of core performance measures to be implemented by 2002. For a detailed discussion of these JCAHO directions and how they will affect your hospital, please read Chapter 3.

Linking your measures to the hospital's strategic goals

Once you've selected all of your measures and ensured that they (1) are mapped to all appropriate JCAHO functions and dimensions of performance, (2) cover each of the JCAHO's required areas, and (3) meet JCAHO's standard benchmarking and ORYX requirements, you're ready to check them to ensure that they are effectively linked to the hospital's strategic goals.

Although this may sound like a complicated task, it is actually quite easy. For example, if the hospital's current goal is to provide better service to the Hispanic community, you can readily target your required patient satisfaction measures to meet it. If your goal is to expand women's services, you might incorporate benchmarked cesarean section rates (which will meet your operative and invasive procedure measurement requirements), neonatal mortality rates (which will measure the JCAHO function of patient treatment), and perhaps patient satisfaction data into your measurement program, thus meeting both the JCAHO's requirements and your own hospital's need for substantive information on performance.

Managing the measurement process
Choosing sample sizes and statistical methods

After you've selected all of the measures that your hospital will conduct, your next important task is to determine how large your sample sizes should be and what statistical methods you will use to manage your measurements. The standards allow you to decide how large the majority of your measurement sample sizes should be. There are only two cases in which a specific sample size is dictated—for the two required measures of operative/invasive procedures review and blood usage review. In each of these instances, the JCAHO requires you to review either 5% of your cases or 30 cases, whichever is smaller.

There is an entire science of sample-size selection, but the 30-case minimum is a good rule to follow whether you're analyzing the JCAHO's required measures or not. You should consult someone competent in statistics if you wish to draw reliable data from a population smaller than 30; and consider seeking advice any time your sample is smaller than 5% as well.

Statistical methods

You should consider using statistical process control (SPC) techniques in at least some instances to help you determine whether performance variations are due to an underlying cause that you can correct or by random events. For example, SPC might be used to evaluate patient satisfaction trends, adverse drug reaction trends, waiting time or result reporting time trends, or complication trends if they are sufficiently frequent in a given population.

The JCAHO has increased its focus on SPC, and surveyors will expect you to explain how the decision was made to use these methods and who assists departments to make the appropriate computations. Expect to receive some surveyor inquiries about whether you considered using SPC to evaluate the quality of some of your performance measures, and be prepared to give examples of how SPC has been used in the organization. (See Bibliography for additional readings on SPC.)

Deciding when and how often to measure

Once you've determined what exactly it is that you must measure, you should decide when and how often it should be measured. Basically, there is no set rule, and you'll have to make that determination based on the nature of the issue you're assessing and the implications of poor performance.

The frequency of measurements must depend on the urgency and magnitude of the problem. For example, if waiting times in the emergency department are a top concern, you should measure them on several shifts weekly to determine if improvements are needed. In a large-volume emergency department, you might be able to collect enough data within 2–3 weeks to support analysis and decision making; in a smaller program it might take longer than 1 month.

If you do identify a problem, you'll need to implement an improvement plan (see Chapters 6 and 12) and, once the improvements have been made, measure the waiting times again (on all pertinent shifts) at least once a month to verify that they have been reduced. Once the waiting times have been stable for a reasonable period and are no longer a major problem, you can stop your measuring altogether.

Remember that measuring is expensive; it carries a direct cost of staff time and energy and an indirect cost of lost opportunities; therefore, it's very important to know when to stop. This does not mean that all stable measures should be discontinued; some should be in place forever as fundamental protections for your patients and staff, such as those that monitor any of the JCAHO-required measurement areas (e.g., infection rates, patient satisfaction, medication errors, or transfusion reactions). However, the frequency with which you measure should be sensitive to the current performance of the hospital: Is this a high-risk and problem-prone area or just a high-volume one? These issues affect how often you conduct these follow-up measurements.

In summary, the frequency of measurement depends on the hospital's current performance levels and resource allocation decision process. There is no simple formula for this, and JCAHO requires only that you be able to explain why you chose to measure at a specific frequency. If you can credibly demonstrate that your decisions were thoughtful and reflected knowledge of the process, national standards, and needs of your patients and other customers, you are likely to have a very positive reaction.

Documenting measurement hospital-wide

Finally, after you've carefully followed all of the JCAHO's measurement requirements and developed a sound set of measures that will help the hospital to improve important processes, you should document exactly what it is that you plan to do. In an ideal world, you could assemble all of the hospital's measures into a single integrated database, cross-reference them to the JCAHO's standards, and show that improvements were implemented by specific teams. But most hospitals do not have this capability and can do a perfectly credible job with ordinary word processing and spreadsheet software packages to document the process and results of performance measurements.

Survey teams generally review your measures as they review PI teams' accomplishments. They will ask the hospital's improvement team how it selected certain measures, how it knew that the collected data were valid and reliable, how it used SPC, and how it assessed the collected data (see Chapter 11).

In addition, the surveyors will ask the hospital's leaders (usually the PI director) to demonstrate that all required measures are in place. If you develop a comprehensive checklist that lists all of your measures and cross-references them to each of the JCAHO's measurement requirements, you'll easily be able to show the surveyors that your measures satisfy the standards. Figure 10.4 shows how to demonstrate compliance with required areas. It does not list *all* of the JCAHO's required measurement areas, because these change from year to year, but it exemplifies the clear documentation you need to prepare confidently for accreditation surveys.

Implementing measures

See Chapters 6 and 7 for much more detail on implementing measurement using individual departments and PI teams.

FIGURE 10.4

Samples of compliance with JCAHO measurement requirements

By mapping the hospital's PI projects to JCAHO functions, you'll be able to demonstrate that the hospital measures its performance in all of the required areas.

Below you'll find a list used in one hospital to prove to surveyors that vigorous PI activity was in place in a wide range of functions. Although this list actually includes only a small fraction of the PI initiatives implemented in the hospital, it was extensive enough to demonstrate to surveyors that the hospital was in full compliance.

Your hospital should compile such a list for surveyors, covering all required measurement areas, perhaps by using Figures 10.1 and 10.2.

Sample JCAHO measurement area[1]	Sample improvement project
Patient rights and organizational ethics	• Improved child protective services processes • Developed confidentiality guidelines • Redesigned the patient satisfaction measurement program
Patient assessment	• Implemented more than 25 clinical paths • Revised blood ordering guidelines

FIGURE 10.4 (cont'd)

Sample JCAHO measurement area[1]	Sample improvement project
Care of patients	• Implemented more than 25 clinical paths • Developed new sedation protocol for ventilated patient in medical intensive care unit • Improved radiology wait times
Operative procedures	• *Patient selection:* Established sinus surgery functional status study • *Patient preparation:* Implemented antibiotic use 2 hours before surgery • *Performance of procedure:* Improved timeliness of operation start times • *Post-procedure and education:* Implemented oxygen therapy and associated patient education for post-anesthesia patients
Medication use	• *Prescribing and ordering:* Ensured that staff comply with antibiotic and albumin guidelines • *Preparing and dispensing:* Monitored medication use errors • *Administering:* Established patient counseling task force • *Monitoring:* Monitored adverse drug reactions
Blood use	• *Ordering, distribution, and handling:* Established specimen collection task force • *Administering:* Implemented patient identification improvement effort • *Monitoring:* Monitored blood transfusion reactions and infectious disease transmission
Performance improvement	• Redesigned the hospital PI process • Investigated all transfusion reactions • Tracked risk management incidents, accidental exposures • Monitored lifting injuries
Leadership	• Developed new strategic plan, redevelopment project, community services plan, and on-site child care program
Environment of care	• Established aspergillus prevention task force • Developed facilities maintenance proactive deployment program • Established neonatal resuscitation resources task force
Human resources	• Redesigned the recruitment process • Improved the timeliness of performance reviews
Information management	• Revised ambulatory surgery preregistration process • Improved the timeliness of laboratory and radiology abnormal values reporting • Established digital dictation system for health information management • Instituted an accounts receivable improvement project
Infection control	• Established a multi–drug-resistant organisms task force • Established a tuberculosis task force • Checked compliance with antibiotics guidelines

[1]Not a comprehensive list of all required areas of measurement.

Chapter 11

Assessing Your Results: Where Do You Go from Here? (PI.4)

Hospital and medical staff leaders often complain that they have "too much data and not enough information." This is why the assessment stage is so critical. By assessing the vast amounts of data gathered by measurement teams, the hospital can transform its data into useful information and determine what improvements should be made.

Without assessment, an improvement effort would be based on mere guesswork, and the hospital would risk significant waste of time, money, energy, and credibility. Therefore, instead of randomly selecting factors to improve, you should fully understand the process in question and its outcomes before you begin to "tinker."

As noted in Chapter 8, every department and performance improvement (PI) team should continually assess its collected data and compare that data to its performance goals. Hospitals should conduct routine monitoring on important measures, such as infection rates, to ensure that performance is within targeted ranges and that intervention is not required. They should also collect data on focused improvement efforts (usually through a team initiative) to collect data to determine whether an improvement has produced the desired results.

The Joint Commission on Accreditation of Healthcare Organizations (JCAHO) has made it abundantly clear that Assessment is an area in which hospitals have not excelled. In fact, in an unprecedented move, the Joint Commission added Assessment to the list of likely random-unannounced-survey focus topics even though it has been extremely rare for surveyors to write Type I recommendations in this area. In other words, although surveyors have been unwilling or unable to cite specific deficiencies in PI Assessment, the JCAHO sees it as one of the most critical problems in hospitals nationally.

How can you respond to this apparent contradiction? Recognize that it can be difficult for a surveyor to write a Type I recommendation for an apparently weak PI Assessment program without strong support and guidance from the JCAHO. That support and guidance seem to be in place now, and in fact the JCAHO's official publications emphasize that, in fact, this will be a significant focus in surveys.

Your best response is to focus on the basics of competent assessment: solid data collection, with due attention to reliability and accuracy; thoughtful statistical analysis (especially statistical process control where appropriate) and careful display of data to support meaningful interpretation; and well-documented discussions of the underlying significance of measurement and the potential implications for action.

Assessment is the link between measurement and action, and indeed it is often a weak link. Measuring is an active process with evident results. Action plans are interesting to develop, and we all want to make change to improve care. The PI Assessment phase, on the other hand, can be slow, maybe confusing, and frustrating, especially if it demonstrates that the problem or opportunity is not as simple as we expected.

As PI director, your job is to prepare for great assessment by ensuring that measurement is solid and by preparing the teams who will assess that data with appropriate education and support. Then they can make meaningful judgments about the data that lead to well-targeted action plans for improvement.

Read through this chapter to learn more about the role of individual departments or PI teams in the assessment phase and how to ensure that these teams conduct their assessments efficiently and in compliance with JCAHO requirements. For more information on how to conduct a hospital-wide self-assessment in which you evaluate the success of your past year's PI program, refer to Chapter 10.

Who conducts assessments?

Most of your hospital's data will be collected by PI teams and assessed by either the PI teams or department managers. Before the teams begin to collect the data, they should develop a plan that states what their goals for measurement and assessment are, such as "showing improvement in a process" or "establishing that at least 80% of patients are seen within 10 minutes of their appointment time." In addition, the teams should understand that they must take that collected data, enter it into an appropriate analytic framework, such as a report, spreadsheet, or graph, and assess the data quarterly, monthly, or weekly, depending on the importance of the issue being measured.

Hospital leaders should also annually assess the quality of the hospital's PI program. In the next chapter, this important process is reviewed in more detail.

Comparing gathered data with JCAHO-required comparative data

As discussed in Chapters 4 and 6, the JCAHO requires hospitals to establish their performance goals in accordance with

- The hospital's past performance
- Other hospitals' performance
- Practice guidelines, parameters, or other current sources
- Customer needs and expectations
- Comparative and reference databases (see also Chapter 3 for information on the new ORYX initiative)

But the standards simply say to "compare your performance"; they don't tell you what comparisons to make, although it is clear that nonclinical processes or procedures do not need to be compared. Surveyors are interested in ensuring that your hospital uses benchmarks and other comparisons to improve patient care. For example, your accounting department, fundraising department, and purchasing functions do not directly affect the quality of patient care, and the JCAHO does not require you to compare them in this way.

Therefore, as you assess gathered data on patient care processes, you should compare them with other organizations' processes, national guidelines, benchmarks, and trends within your own hospital. For example, a team working to improve the speed of admissions from the emergency department should match its results against data on this process from other hospitals or from literature on best practices. These comparisons will help the team to determine how the hospital's process matches up against the performance of similar groups. But remember that although these comparisons offer your hospital valuable information and data, not every measure you take must be compared to outside benchmarks. You need to conduct only some comparisons to meet JCAHO requirements.

Once all of the data on the hospital's own performance and comparative performance measures at other organizations have been collected, a department manager or the PI team will sit down and analyze it all. In many cases, special analytic tools will be needed to determine whether significant changes have been made. You might use the JCAHO's recommended statistical process control tool to analyze the data, or you might use other statistical tools such as t-tests or changes in coefficients of variation.

Whoever analyzes the data should always keep in mind that assessment is more than a simple statistical portrait of your gathered data. Assessment involves interpretation. One way to ensure that your data have been thoughtfully assessed in accordance with JCAHO standards is to ask yourself the following three questions as you analyze each indicator:

- How are we performing on this indicator compared to our goal?

- If we have improved the process and met our goal, do the statistics and our own knowledge confirm that the change is stable, genuine, and reliably producing the desired performance? Or do we need additional time to confirm that the process is stable?

- If we have not met our target yet, why haven't we? Based on data and observation, what contributed to our less-than-targeted performance? If we don't know exactly what factors these were, what can we do in the coming period to collect more complete data?

Identifying sentinel events and "bad apples"

The JCAHO also requires you to assess two important types of events: (1) "important single events," often called *sentinel events*; and (2) individual performance failures, or what might colloquially be called *bad apples*.

Sentinel events
Sentinel events are "important single events," such as an error or lack of judgment that caused, or potentially could have caused, a serious and unexpected negative outcome. This negative outcome could be a complication requiring a change in medical treatment, a death, or even a narrowly averted problem that revealed the potential for serious harm. Sentinel events would include chemotherapy errors or perhaps a significant breach in infection control.

Chapter 11

Hospitals must assess sentinel events, including at least

- Discrepancies between preoperative and postoperative diagnoses
- Adverse events during anesthesia
- Confirmed transfusion reactions
- Significant adverse drug reactions

The objective is to prevent recurrence of the event by examining the underlying systems that contributed to the error (if any) and looking for opportunities for improvement.

Beyond the types of incidents described above, the JCAHO does not prescribe specifically which sentinel events should be addressed in your PI process. It is up to each hospital to establish criteria and systems to identify which "important single events" should be the focus of a PI team. Within the hospital, each unit or department may have somewhat different criteria. A cardiac arrest in a coronary care unit would not be a sentinel event in most cases; but a cardiac arrest in a psychiatry unit probably would be, and it should be evaluated to ensure that patient assessment was appropriate.

You should use your hospital's information management system to help you identify all sentinel events. For example, your hospital should require all patient care and support areas to discuss recent sentinel events (per their own definitions) at all department meetings. The focus of the review is on whether the event may have been prevented and whether preparation to handle it may have been more effective if hospital systems and resources had been organized differently.

The JCAHO prescribes "intensive assessment" of these "important single events." See Figure 10.4 for an overview of the JCAHO's sentinel event policy. If management and medical leadership believe that there may have been a way to improve the handling of the situation, they may wish to form a formal PI team to examine the issue from a more comprehensive perspective. They should certainly charter PI teams to review the systems involved in highly important sentinel events. For example, a single occurrence of a retained surgical sponge may simply warrant an audit of counting procedures and postsurgical patient monitoring, especially if the problem was identified promptly and the patient treated quickly. On the other hand, the amputation of the wrong limb could appropriately warrant an extremely intensive review of procedures, communications, training, and documentation in the surgical process, as well as a thorough review of competence and performance of each individual involved in the process.

Accreditation watch

In mid-1996, the JCAHO announced a new initiative to conduct unannounced and unsolicited visits to hospitals in which "adverse sentinel events" came to the attention of the JCAHO. The stated purpose of this new program is to ensure a formal review of systems and procedures in hospitals involved in serious events that posed a potential threat to patient care. The policy was revised and clarified early in 1997.

An "adverse sentinel event" is "an unexpected occurrence involving death or serious physical or psychological injury or the risk thereof [and] specifically includes loss of limb or function."

Several hospitals have experienced this review and have indicated that it focused (1) on whether the hospital paid serious attention to developing a credible "root-cause analysis" of the systems and individual performance issues involved in high-profile errors such as a chemotherapy error and (2) whether management devoted appropriate resources to correcting these issues.

JCAHO has created a status of "accreditation watch" to be imposed in such a situation, which would continue until the hospital has demonstrated that the underlying problems have been addressed. The origin of this new status is to be found in some of the criticism of JCAHO from Public Citizen and other organizations that believe the accrediting agency is insufficiently tough on hospitals with widely publicized quality problems.

Apprehension about a potential JCAHO "accreditation watch" should never be the sole, or even a primary, motivation for a hospital to address observed system and performance problems. However, as JCAHO continues to pursue this process, it is likely to generate information and insight that will be helpful to all hospitals seeking to address these problems promptly and appropriately.

Generally, transfusion reactions, adverse drug reactions, and postoperative diagnosis discrepancies (typically related to pathology) are assessed through standing management and committee processes, but they also depend on good information flow through risk management and medical records. For example, a blood transfusion committee, the pharmacy and therapeutics committee, and the appropriate surgical quality committee will assess sentinel events in these respective areas. But they need to know when issues arise. Data collection through incident reports, pharmacy records (e.g., when medications are ordered to reverse an adverse drug reaction), and pathology data, as well as routine medical record screening and evaluation of patient complaints, will be needed to identify these events so that the committees can review them.

"Bad apples"

Traditional quality assurance is almost universally, though perhaps unfairly, described as "the theory of bad apples" because traditional quality assurance focuses on poor individual performance rather than systems failures as the source of quality problems. The JCAHO recognizes that individual performance can indeed contribute to poor quality; therefore, it requires your hospital to identify such situations and deal appropriately with individuals who perform poorly, whether they are members of the medical staff (MS.4.3.3) or other employees or contractors (LD.2.1.5, HR.4).

The key here is to measure appropriately and to ensure that the necessary data are being collected to display outcomes according to individual practitioners. This information will help you to determine whether individual performance varies notably. For instance, the radiology department might collect information on the specific radiographer involved with each image and periodically compare image quality across individuals. If the department does not collect this information in the first place, each radiologist's performance cannot be objectively assessed.

If an individual performance problem is identified, according to the MS, LD, and HR standards the hospital must counsel, retrain, and perhaps discipline the individual, while restricting his or her clinical privileges and activity as necessary to ensure that patient care is not jeopardized.

Documenting assessments

Documenting the assessment process within an individual department or PI team is a byproduct of the group's work. Surveyors will review documents such as data displays, tables, and graphs as well as departmental and governing board meeting minutes to determine whether you

- Interpreted data accumulated during the measurement process
- Discussed whether more intensive assessments were warranted
- Reviewed data to determine whether important processes were stable
- Evaluated whether the process under review met the hospital's needs

Through a hierarchy of reporting (Figure 11.1), assessment results should be evaluated as appropriate by department managers and other senior leaders in the hospital. A small group of critical indicators should be ultimately submitted to the governing board for periodic review (see the following section for more information on assessment reporting). A typical report on the assessment of a quality measure should include

- A description of the measure, why it is important, and which JCAHO functions and dimensions are being evaluated
- The time frame of the data reflected in the report
- The target value for the measure, or target performance of this process
- Current period data and trend data over time
- A discussion of the implications of the data (e.g., we are within our target range and believe its stable performance because it's been within the target range for four measuring periods; we're not within our target range but think we're close because we've had statistically significant improvement over the past three quarters; or performance has declined due to turnover, and there's a need for retraining)
- Your findings and conclusions describing what interventions, if any, are needed
- A description of the next steps (e.g., continue to measure, assign priority for improvement, discontinue or decrease frequency of measurement, and communicate with affected groups)

Reporting your results to the quality oversight committee

When the hospital developed its PI plan, it determined which issues were high priorities and should be monitored by the quality oversight committee (see Chapter 5). This committee should globally monitor and keep track of the hospital's major priorities for the year. It should also regularly review important indicators, such as adverse drug reactions, infection rates, lengths of stay, or complications, even if these issues are not specifically targeted for improvement at present.

PI teams working on improving key processes or collecting important data should report their assessments of the collected data to the oversight committee for its review on a regular basis. In addition, it is advisable to report data every quarter on consistently high-profile measures for your hospital, such as patient satisfaction, turnaround time in computed tomography, or infection rates, even if they are well under control. The quality oversight committee will also want to review data on all important newly designed patient care processes. For instance, implementation of a new solid-organ transplant program may warrant regular reports on complications, mortality, and patient satisfaction in this group for the first couple of years.

FIGURE 11.1

Reporting hierarchy

In the PI plan, you will define reporting structures so that the assessment of data is communicated appropriately. A typical structure might include the following:

Each department

- Establishes routine monitoring indicators
- Selects a limited number of improvement priorities consistent with hospital-wide priorities and according to defined authorization approaches
- Selects key highlights each month or so and reports them via management representative to the quality oversight committee

Quality oversight committee

- Based on the annual plan, provides agenda time and focus on selected monitoring indicators
- Receives routine reports on all major improvement projects
- Selects key highlights each month and reports on them via management representative to the board of directors

Board of directors

- Reviews a concise group of important monitoring indicators (e.g., infection rate)
- Reviews progress at intervals on a small group of key improvement priorities
- Reviews major improvement programs comprehensively at appropriate intervals

In establishing this reporting hierarchy, you want to ensure that each level receives as much data as necessary (and no more) to perform its stewardship and leadership functions. Excessive reporting results in committees that drown in details and don't have sufficient perspective to make resource decisions. In addition, you should remember that inadequate reporting fails to meet JCAHO and common sense requirements for effective leadership.

Less important issues can be left to individual departments for monitoring and assessment. For example, if waiting time is under control in a department but is still monitored regularly because it is important to patients, you do not need to report this information to the hospital's quality committee. An annual mention of the indicator in the department's self-assessment (see Chapter 12) may suffice.

Conducting the hospital-wide performance improvement assessment

It is necessary that every hospital undertake a thorough annual self-assessment of its PI program. This would be appropriate even in the absence of JCAHO standards because the principle of PI is to monitor and examine performance in search of opportunities for improvement.

More specifics on this hospital-wide assessment process are found in Chapter 12.

Notes

Chapter 12

The Final Stage: Implementing Improvements (PI.5)

As noted previously, both the Joint Commission on Accreditation of Healthcare Organizations (JCAHO) and hospital leaders are well aware that hospitals will find many more opportunities for improvement than can be realistically improved. In fact, they fully expect that you can identify some opportunities that you did *not* pursue in a given year. Therefore, hospitals should focus their energies on those improvements that are genuinely important to patient care and represent a cost benefit appropriate to the hospital's community.

In the performance improvement (PI) standards, the JCAHO explicitly outlines how hospitals should set their PI priorities and use their finances and human resources. Specifically, the PI.5 standards require hospitals to demonstrate that they

- Are aware of a range of opportunities for improvement, based on routine and special monitors and measurements.
- Select appropriate, high-priority processes for improvement.
- Perform the PI cycle ("plan, design, measure, assess, improve," or comparable) competently.
- Show actual, sustained improvement in processes designated for improvement. Those that have not shown sustained improvement need your attention: specifically, a documented discussion producing a set of practical goals and an action plan for getting back on track.

In addition, you should make it a priority to demonstrate that your hospital has improvement activities or at least measurement and monitoring activities going on in all 11 of the JCAHO's functional areas. Although measurement in the 11 functional areas is no longer specifically stated as a requirement, the JCAHO recommends that, as a logical starting point, the leaders should review the important functions common to all healthcare organizations identified by the primary chapter titles in the *Comprehensive Accreditation Manual for Hospitals* (*CAMH*). If you have no monitoring in place, it will be difficult to demonstrate that you have reviewed these functions. In most hospitals, it should not be difficult to ensure that there is some relevant activity in each of these 11 areas, as they are indeed fundamental to successful patient care operations.

Read through this chapter to learn how to improve your processes in accordance with JCAHO requirements and how to document your compliance both for individual PI teams and the hospital as a whole.

Chapter 12

Establishing your improvement priorities

After you've determined what areas you should measure and have collected and analyzed the resulting data, you will probably develop a long list of processes that need improvement. For example, you may find that infection rates are high in a particular area, that radiology turnaround time for computed tomography scan reports is double what it was a year ago (angering attending physicians as well as patients), that errors on patient bills are causing insurance denials, and that patients are unhappy with the food! Ideally, every hospital would like to address and improve each of its identified problem areas, but, most hospitals do not have the time, resources, or manpower to implement such a wide array of improvement projects.

The JCAHO understands this dilemma and does not expect you to improve every single problem you uncover. You'll meet surveyors' expectations as long as you assess your measurement data, identify the hospital's areas of poor performance, and then determine which of these trouble spots needs immediate attention based on management's assessments of patient and community needs.

In this context, pay special attention to the national crusade against medical errors. Even if your own hospital's data do not indicate that you have a high-priority problem in medication errors, surgical side selection, competence for procedures, etc., you and other hospital leaders are your community's champions in maintaining the highest standards of sound healthcare. It is evident that the JCAHO, Health Care Financing Administration, and other regulatory agencies do not believe that hospitals have put in place reliable measurement and improvement activities sufficient to reduce medical error. It is critical that you are working at the very least to improve data collection on errors and to study potential trends. Consult references such as the *Institute for Safe Medication Practices* and others (see Bibliography) for high-profile opportunities.

The minutes of your quality oversight committee meeting should clearly document the results of your assessments and describe why the committee selected each improvement priority. The minutes should also document which measures will require future monitoring.

Remember that any measurement data revealing a real and significant risk to patient safety or care should not be ignored. If there are patterns of medication errors, an increase in patient adverse outcomes, or any measure that reasonably indicates that patient well-being is threatened, JCAHO surveyors will expect to see that you have researched and addressed the problem appropriately and promptly.

Approaches to priority setting: explicit or implicit?
The following is a brief review of two approaches to setting improvement priorities. Both approaches have advantages and disadvantages. The explicit approach is excellent for highly disciplined, goal-directed organizations, but it can yield some rigidity and can mean that new opportunities cannot be promptly seized. The implicit approach is suitable for less formal cultures but may fail to bring resources together effectively in a disciplined and forceful manner to address problems and bring them to closure. Many organizations use a mixture of both approaches. In any case, it is important for JCAHO compliance that you be able to document and demonstrate that priorities are set consciously by an appropriately authorized and chartered group, typically the quality oversight committee.

Surveyors will ask you to discuss your process for setting priorities. Some hospitals have reported an enthusiastic surveyor reaction to highly formalized and explicit approaches (e.g., numeric ranking of importance of factors in PI, followed by multivoting and ranking each proposed PI project). However, the standards do not require such a formal approach, and you can achieve compliance as long as the approach you do use, even an implicit and consensus-based one, is documented and followed.

But whether you take an explicit or implicit approach to priority setting, you must perform the selection of priorities carefully and document the selection process completely. To fulfill the JCAHO's standards of leadership and PI and to focus resources where they are likely to make the most difference, you should be sure to

- Charter teams strategically, where their efforts make a real difference
- Focus on areas with mature and constructive medical staff relationships
- Focus on areas with mature and sophisticated management
- Select priorities based on solid comparative performance information

Read through the following information to learn more about explicit and implicit priority setting and to help you decide which method would work best in your organization.

Setting explicit priorities for improvement

One approach to priority setting is to use a formal, top-down, explicit priority-setting process anchored in the annual PI plan's goals.

First, your quality committee should review the hospital's annual PI plan and refresh itself on the organization's key priorities for the upcoming year. This serves two purposes. Reviewing the priorities of the PI plan will help the committee identify potential improvement projects that will further the hospital's overall PI goals. In addition, the committee can examine the progress of ongoing projects to make sure improvement is sustained, as required by the JCAHO.

For example, if your organization's top priorities this year are to improve patient satisfaction with the emergency department, implement a cardiac surgery program, and improve pathology services, you should select improvement projects that will complement those objectives (e.g., reduce waiting time and improve patient communications in the emergency department). You may also find that you have the energy and resources to address other priorities (e.g., reduce waiting time and improve patient communication in ambulatory surgery), but those should be second in line for attention.

Next, the committee should charter formal PI teams (see Chapter 7) to address the highest-priority and most complex interdepartmental and interdisciplinary processes, such as inpatient admissions from the emergency department, blood management in the operating room, or stat specimen reporting cycle times. Other goals proposed during the year for PI are evaluated against key hospital-wide goals and may be deferred or denied if they do not substantively advance them. For example, perhaps a manager has proposed a priority for speeding up the turnaround time on stat complete blood cell count results for the emergency department. Although that seems to be a helpful goal, the committee may think that the emergency department and laboratory managers can perform some measurement together and then come back with a more elaborated proposal based on specific data. Or the committee may think that the laboratory has other priorities this year that are even more critical and that this issue will have to wait until those are addressed.

As discussed in Chapter 5, the quality committee and senior managers may need to make difficult decisions at times. Even when the data demonstrate that an area is not performing as well as you might like, it might be necessary to delay improvement efforts in that area if other priorities are more pressing, if resources are simply unavailable, if the area's personnel are not sufficiently stable because of recent management changes or high turnover, or for other reasons.

If the committee cannot reach consensus on key priorities, even based on the year's PI plan, then formal group process techniques, such as multivoting and prioritization matrices, may be useful (see Bibliography). All of these steps should be documented accurately for use during the JCAHO survey.

Setting priorities for improvement with implicit criteria

Another and perhaps more common approach to priority setting is to use a less formal implicit priority-setting process based on consensus among quality oversight committee members.

Using this model for new projects, the hospital's quality committee will continuously consider potential improvement projects identified through means such as formal quality reporting, referrals from the medical executive committee, and so on. For example, when the decision is made to implement a new cardiac surgery program, the committee will determine which quality measures should be implemented at the same time, then it will work with each department to integrate these measures and decide which older and less productive measures should be retired to free up time and energy for the new program. As other important initiatives come to the committee's attention, the readjustment of priorities will continue.

Designing your improvement plan

Once you've performed your assessments and selected your improvement priorities, it will be time to begin the most rewarding, and the most difficult, component of PI: designing process changes to yield improved performance.

The literature on working with teams describes many approaches to constructing better processes: brainstorming, benchmarking, quality function deployment, design of experiments, etc. (see Chapters 7 and 8). But no matter which approach you take, the basic strategy is still the same. To make improvements, a PI team will need to completely rethink the process in question.

The team working on the design will produce in most cases a flow chart, a narrative, and supporting data and documents such as job descriptions, budget requests, and benchmark analyses, which together will define a new approach to producing the desired results. This design will go back to relevant managers for their approval and an allocation of resources, typically for a pilot-testing phase. (See Chapter 7 for a discussion of improvement teams that cannot break through to an improved process design or that cannot do so at an acceptable cost.)

Implementing improvements

The JCAHO's standards, and virtually all commonly used PI methodologies (see Chapter 5), require hospitals to pilot-test planned improvements wherever feasible and to conduct data-based evaluations of the pilot tests before implementing any permanent changes to a process.

For example, if a team working on improving admission times from the emergency department plans to recommend the distribution of pagers to patient transportation staff, it might test this plan out for a couple of weeks and collect careful data on the results before investing in a whole new set of pagers. Or if the team plans to suggest that the emergency department should employ its own transporter, it might reassign someone to this function for a while to gauge if this is a good solution, rather than hire a new position right away. Another approach is to test the proposed improvement on one patient care floor but not on another and to use the unchanged floor as a "control group" or comparison (this has been used for clinical pathways in some instances). Or, some improvements could be tested on alternate days or shifts. For a highly detailed and quantitative approach to testing changed processes, consult the literature on design of experiments (see Bibliography); while relatively little has been done in this area in healthcare, there have been some case studies, and the methodology has some applicability.

Most often, a pilot test in a complex hospital environment tends to be time-based: Try the new method for a period, collect performance data carefully, and evaluate whether an improvement has been achieved.

During the pilot test, gathered data may indicate that the new process has introduced a new type of problem, complication, or issue. The team should monitor the data closely to catch such an undesirable finding quickly and to determine whether the change should be reversed immediately or whether further fine-tuning is needed. For instance, if a clinical pathway is implemented and it is quickly observed that patients are being readmitted more frequently, the pathway will probably be suspended while the cause of the readmissions is evaluated carefully. On the other hand, if a new system of food tray delivery is implemented and a higher rate of employee injuries from the new carts is observed, retraining and observation may be a more reasonable solution to the problem than reverting to the old system. On some occasions, an improvement will be found to be effective but may cost more than expected, and this will require evaluation and balancing of priorities as well.

When surveyors visit your hospital, they'll want to see specific examples of improvement efforts that were implemented after pilot testing and to learn about any refinements you made to the process as a result of the pilot test. And if a decision is made late in the improvement effort to cancel or defer implementation of the new process, documentation should be maintained to describe the rationale for the decision. As with other improvement-related decisions, the JCAHO expects that the rationale will be related directly to the hospital's mission and priorities and that resources are available.

During the improvement phase, the team will need to remain well-focused on the action plan to ensure that real progress is being made on real objectives; it is easy to become drawn into a tangent or a "fun" enhancement, although the core improvement needed by your patients requires some tough decisions and turf battles to be resolved! Stringent, continuous focus on the team's original objectives and action plan will need to be enforced. The quality director can help keep the group on target through monitoring minutes and requesting periodic updates on progress (Figure 12.1; to match PI projects to JCAHO requirements, see Figure 10.2, page 139).

Documenting your actions

To demonstrate compliance with the improvement (PI.5) standards to surveyors, you must produce a variety of documents that describe

Chapter 12

- Which performance problems you identified
- How you planned to remedy them
- Whether your efforts were successful

Often, your PI teams' workbooks can offer surveyors just this type of evidence. For example, a typical team's workbook is likely to include documents that cover the full scope of the PI process, from planning to implementing improvements (Figure 12.2). Many such workbooks include the following:

- Plan: a memo requesting the team members' participation, sent by the sponsoring individual or committee and incorporating the team charter statement; summaries of the team's analysis of the current process through data collected and assessments of the data (perhaps documented in the minutes); and minutes of all team meetings

- Design: minutes describing how the team redesigned the process; summaries of process changes made, perhaps documented by new policies and procedures or new flow charts

- Measure: documents describing the collected data

- Assess: analysis and assessment of the effectiveness of the changes made to the process

- Improve: minutes describing the team's success (e.g., did we actually change the process to produce improvement?)

In addition, well-designed storyboards or posters succinctly summarizing a team's work can demonstrate to a surveyor that your organization knows how to improve its performance in full compliance with the standards. (Figure 12.3.) A few storyboards can tell surveyors a lot about your organization: your culture of PI; the multidisciplinary nature of your teams; the breadth and depth of your knowledge about statistics, measurement, and assessment; and the meaningfulness of your projects. By highlighting actual PI projects and their results, these storyboards will help you to prove that your PI process really works.

Documenting the hospital's PI results can be a tedious and time-consuming task, and in a busy hospital it may be difficult to persuade staff to take the time to formally document what they've accomplished. Therefore, it's up to you to overcome this hurdle by recognizing and rewarding employees who correctly document the results of their improvement projects and by implementing various systems that motivate staff to document their PI activities properly.

Annual performance improvement poster events

Many hospitals hold annual PI poster events to encourage PI teams to document their improvement results properly. At these events, PI teams present storyboards covering their work. These events are fun, but they are not required for JCAHO compliance. If you do decide to hold a PI poster event, you can go about it in many different ways, depending on your hospital's culture and preference.

Poster days take a fair amount of staff work in logistics, and they take time for PI teams to develop posters, but they are a wonderful way to show employees and physicians what excellent improvements are being made, to teach them about PI concepts, and to provide reward and recognition for team members. As you plan to set up your own poster day, you should ask yourself:

- Should participation be voluntary or mandatory? If you decide to use the posters as a way to demonstrate compliance with surveyors, you may need to make participation

FIGURE 12.1

Performance improvement team progress report

Name of improvement project:

Description of project:

PI team leader:

PI team members:

Original project completion date:

Revised project completion date:

Describe current progress:

What are the key measures the team has adopted for evaluating its progress?

Measure	Performance goal	Current level of performance
1.		
2.		
3.		
4.		
5.		

General comments on the team's progress:

Chapter 12

FIGURE 12.2

Performance improvement team workbook contents

Each team engaged in creating or revising a process should maintain a workbook containing the following elements:

Initial team charter and membership

Minutes of all meetings

Outlines of team educational sessions

Work plan as it is developed and revised over time

Specifically defined goals for the revised process: measurable process and outcome metrics, which are expected to change

Significant work products (cause and effect studies, important data collection summaries, benchmarking or major literature, guidelines, or standards)

Copies of formal recommendations to other committees or leaders

Copies of educational programs, process or policy changes, or other evidence of how the proposed change was implemented, and whether it was pilot tested or not

Data from pilot tests and documented findings and conclusions from the tests

Data from final process change implementation

Evaluation of success of the change based on the planned metrics

Documentation of team discussion, including memoranda and referrals to other committees or leadership, to assure that the change will be maintained and monitored periodically

---

mandatory, at least for those teams working on the annual PI priorities for the hospital.

- Should we label each poster with the pertinent JCAHO "functions"? If you assign each poster to one or more of the 11 required JCAHO functional categories, you will achieve several goals—you'll ensure that you have ongoing PI in all necessary areas, educate staff about what those categories are, and offer opportunities for recognition in each of the 11 categories.

- Should we establish a "core format" for the poster design? You will be well advised to encourage staff to use a consistent core format that is linked to your PI methodology. This will make the posters easier to understand and will also help educate staff further about the importance of following the approved methodology.

FIGURE 12.3

Sample presentation

This presentation demonstrates how we used the plan, do, check, act model to design and implement an improvement in our systems for care of the latex-sensitive patient.

Slide 1: PLAN—Background

- Prevalence of latex sensitivity is increasing
- Our environment and work force need to be prepared to provide safe and effective care for latex-sensitive patients
- Standardized "Latex Sensitivity Cart" developed and implemented [date], including supplies and educational materials for staff
- Continued improvement was needed

Slide 2: PLAN—Objective

- Improve consistency and safety of our systems for identification and care of latex-sensitive patients

Slide 3: PLAN—Action Plan

- Improve patient assessment and identification
- Continue to enhance the standard latex-free cart with commonly needed supplies and reference/educational material for staff
- Enhance crash cart safety for latex-sensitive patients
- Improve staff education on use of latex sensitivity resources

Slide 4: DO—Identification

- Implement use of 'isolation' field by admitting/registration staff
- Enhance communications with nursing unit

Slide 5: DO—Crash Carts

- Replace items with latex where feasible
- Label remaining items clearly

Slide 6: DO—Staff Education

- Creation of staff "Alert" on latex sensitivity
- Unit added to annual Health & Safety training curriculum
- Included info at Safety Fair, [date]

Slide 7: DO—Other

- Integrated into redevelopment planning
- Improved integration with Occupational Latex Exposure task force

Slide 8: CHECK

- Utilization of latex-free cart
- Monitoring of successful patient care: absence of problems; good patient satisfaction
- Identification of further opportunities for improvement

Chapter 12

FIGURE 12.3 (cont'd)

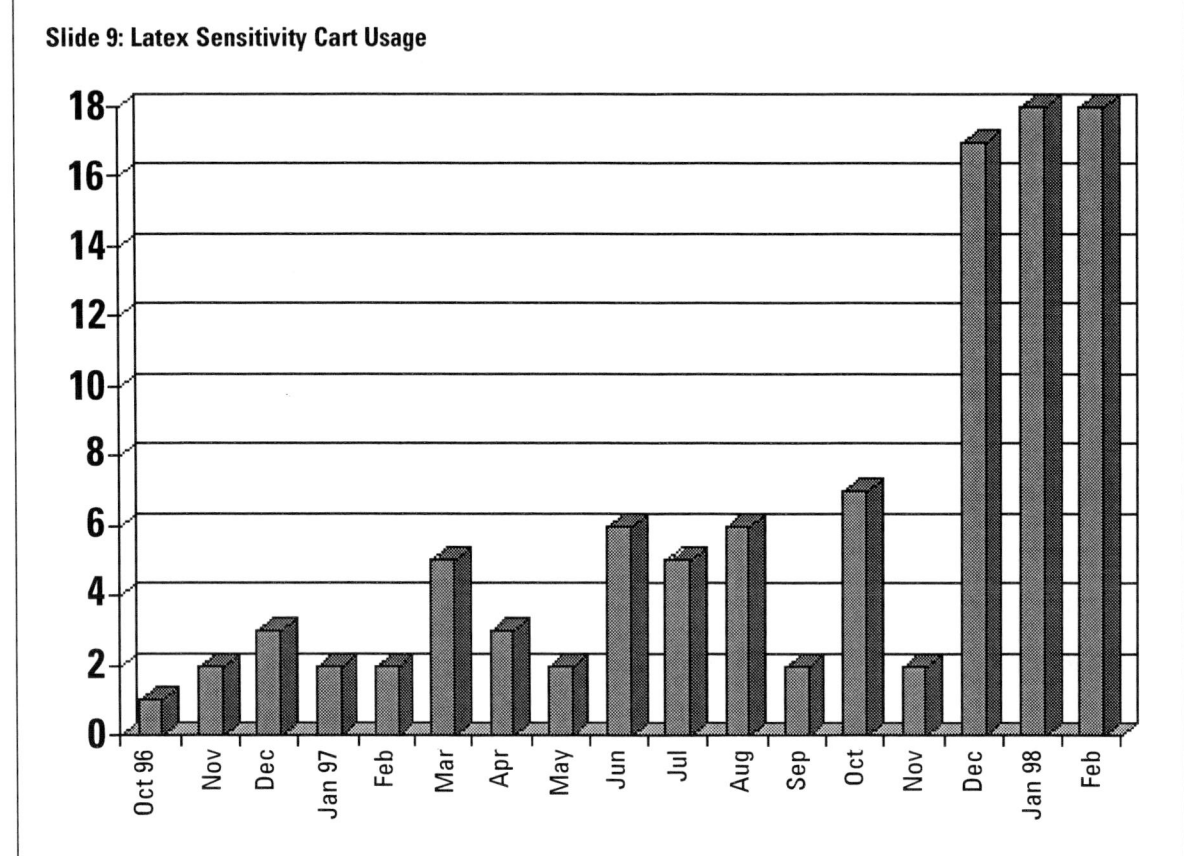

Slide 9: Latex Sensitivity Cart Usage

[Bar chart showing values from Oct 96 through Feb 98, y-axis 0 to 18]

Graph shows number of carts ordered per month

Slide 10: ACT—Next Steps

- Finalize policies/procedures, ensure consistent usage throughout
- Integrate new product labelling mandated by FDA
- Continue to monitor program and evolving knowledge as well as new products
- Develop more sophisticated screening for type and extent of sensitivity to improve efficiency

- Should we hold evaluations to identify the "best" posters? You may want the quality oversight committee or management and medical leadership to judge the best posters, perhaps in each of the JCAHO functional categories. Again, this will help educate staff and reinforce the importance of PI in the minds of all attendees. You may alternatively, or also, want to offer everyone who attends the poster day a chance to vote on their own favorites. This encourages staff to examine each poster more closely and really consider the strengths and merits of the projects.

- Should we offer prizes or other forms of recognition? This will depend on your budget for both time and money, but some form of recognition event (even if it is simply incorporated as another agenda item in an existing management and medical leaders' meeting) is a wonderful way to emphasize the importance of PI for the organization.

All submitted storyboards should include the team members' names and the departments to which they belong. They should also reflect the hospital's PI methodology. For example, if your hospital uses the PDCA (*p*lan, *d*o, *c*heck, *a*ct) model, then each storyboard should include information such as

- **Plan** What was the team's improvement plan? How was it developed?
- **Do** What major changes did the team implement? What did the changes cost? How long did it take to implement them? Were they implemented on a pilot basis first?
- **Check** How did the team ensure that its changes really resulted in improved performance? Which measures improved? How significant were the improvements?
- **Act** How did the team implement the change after the pilot test? How will the team monitor the changes to ensure that the process remains improved?

These posters are an excellent example of compliance with the PI standards and should be displayed prominently during your JCAHO survey. For example, one hospital exhibited all 40 of its most recent posters in a large conference room during the document review session on the first morning of its survey. The surveyors reviewed the posters at lunchtime, and once they were finished, the hospital moved the posters back to their respective departments to allow the surveyors to examine them more closely during their department visits. This approach was very well received by the surveyors; they thought that it allowed them to rapidly review the scope of the PI program and ensure that

- The hospital implemented multidisciplinary improvement projects in many different areas, not just in departments such as nursing or pharmacy
- The hospital's PI methodology was widely used and understood
- Staff improved patient care meaningfully using concrete performance data

The same hospital also published a booklet of brief abstracts of the poster projects each year, so that the JCAHO team could quickly review a broad scope of projects for 3 years at a time to see the depth and solidity of the PI program.

Conducting the annual hospital-wide appraisal

To demonstrate full compliance with the JCAHO's PI.5 standard, the hospital must assess and evaluate how successful its PI program has been. Basically, this entails determining whether you

- Conducted a competent PI program that covered all required areas and activities
- Actually effected improvement in ways that matter to your patients and other customers, according to your annual PI plan

The best way to approach this is to conduct ongoing reviews of the work of each PI team and each departmental PI effort. You'll need to establish that these groups did indeed perform the PI process well and that everyone in the hospital worked together well to implement improvements. Ideally, individual departments and teams should evaluate their own progress and success periodically (Figure 12.4 provides a sample checklist). These reviews should be passed on to the hospital's quality director, who will monitor them, along with all other committee reports and minutes and other processes and products as they are developed, taking note of which items fulfill the JCAHO's requirements particularly well (see Chapters 6 and 7). When new to PI, departments or teams will benefit from relatively frequent self-assessment (perhaps quarterly). As they mature and begin to perform this process almost automatically through the year, a twice-yearly formal review may be sufficient.

FIGURE 12.4

Performance improvement team and departmental self-assessment

Directions: As you conduct the hospital-wide self-assessment, you'll need to determine how well individual PI teams and departments improved the hospital's processes. Ask PI team leaders and department managers to complete the following checklist after they have completed a PI project. The information you gather will help you decide whether your PI program is truly on track.

Name of improvement project: _____

Department(s) involved: _____

Completed by: _____ Date: _____

Developing the performance improvement plan

Yes   No

❑   ❑   Did you follow the hospital's PI model as you analyzed problems and improvement opportunities?

❑   ❑   Did you work with your staff/PI team to identify opportunities for PI?

Designing processes

If you designed a new process:

Yes   No

❑   ❑   Did you clearly and explicitly link it to our mission?

❑   ❑   Did you use the hospital's PI model to ensure that you considered all relevant factors and approached problem solving and design consistent with the hospital's approach?

❑   ❑   Did you explicitly consider the needs, expectations, ideas, and preferences of patients and other customers?

❑   ❑   Did you use up-to-date benchmarks, guidelines, and professional literature as resources?

❑   ❑   Did you study how the process works and what results it produces in other organizations (comparative databases, surveys, etc.)?

If you worked to revise a process:

Yes   No

❑   ❑   Did you clearly define all stages of the process (e.g., when it starts and stops, who are its customers, what JCAHO functions and dimensions of performance it applies to)?

❑   ❑   Did you determine why improvement of this process is important to your customers at this time and why/how it is in sync with the hospital's strategic plan and mission?

❑   ❑   Did you involve relevant departments/disciplines besides your own in the improvement process?

❑   ❑   Did you make this improvement project a priority to ensure that staff have the time and resources to implement improvements?

Conducting measurements

Yes   No

❑   ❑   Did you follow your PI plan as developed?

❑   ❑   Did you measure high-volume, high-risk, and/or problem-prone activities?

❑   ❑   Did you assess patient and other customer satisfaction regularly?

FIGURE 12.4 (cont'd)

❏	❏	As appropriate to the process you were investigating, did you measure JCAHO-required areas, such as the quality of
❏	❏	– Operative and invasive procedures?
❏	❏	– Medication use?
❏	❏	– Blood use?
❏	❏	– Utilization management?
❏	❏	– Behavior management procedures?
❏	❏	– Autopsy results?
❏	❏	– Risk management?
❏	❏	– Quality control in the laboratory, diagnostic radiology, food and nutrition, nuclear medicine, radiation oncology, and equipment used to prepare and administer medication?

Analyzing data and processes

Yes No

❏	❏	Did you analyze your data according to your PI plan?
❏	❏	Did you review the gathered data to see if the process is consistently meeting desired targets/thresholds/goals (i.e., the process is a stable process and not just achieving the goal on average)?
❏	❏	Did you evaluate results of actions taken last month or last quarter to see whether they had the desired effect?
❏	❏	Did you use statistical quality control techniques when appropriate, such as sampling, control charts, or analysis of standard deviations or other measures of variability?
❏	❏	Did you trend your quality data over time?
❏	❏	Did you bring in information from professional literature, benchmarks, comparative databases, practice parameters, guidelines, and so on as you evaluated your processes and outcomes?
❏	❏	If you saw that a process produced inconsistent or undesirable results, did you study it more intensively?
❏	❏	Did you use sentinel events to identify processes needing improvement, without focusing unnecessarily on truly one-time problems that were unrelated to processes?

Evaluating improvements

Yes No

❏	❏	Can you demonstrate that you improved the quality of your process? Or do you have proper measures in place to help you evaluate the process over time?
❏	❏	When appropriate, do you make sure that data gathered during quality studies is used to help evaluate and counsel employees for better performance?
❏	❏	Do you conduct pilot tests of modified processes when appropriate?
❏	❏	Do you focus improvement efforts on processes rather than on individual performance?

Communicating performance improvement information

Yes No

❏	❏	Do you share information on the progress of PI activities with all staff every month?
❏	❏	Do you regularly solicit staff views on opportunities for improvement?
❏	❏	Do you regularly coordinate PI activities with medical leadership and feel sure that there are vehicles to share information about progress with medical staff who use your services/unit?
❏	❏	For support services, do you share information about quality improvement with your customers?

Chapter 12

FIGURE 12.5

Request for information on annual performance improvement achievements

The following is a sample request you can use to solicit a summary of departments' key accomplishments during the year. This gathered information will yield the raw data you'll need to develop the hospital's annual PI assessment.

To: **All Managers**
     All Medical Leadership

From: **Performance Improvement Director**

We are preparing our annual PI report, highlighting specific improvements in quality of care and service that have been achieved through our PI efforts (including clinical paths and other team efforts) during the past year. This report is required by our board and is part of our JCAHO compliance documentation as well. It is an opportunity to recognize the outstanding work being done throughout our organization to improve quality through processes and outcomes that matter to patients and others.

We'd appreciate it if you would take a moment to make a list of the top three or more PI achievements made in your department over the past year. For example, we would like to know

- What was the process (or outcome) that you improved?
- Whether the improvement has been completed or is still under way.
- Which departments were involved.

This request applies to *all* departments, not only the clinical and patient support areas.

Please note that achievements should be articulated in quantitative form when possible. For instance, "98% of patients achieved such and such an outcome, an improvement from 88% in [year], and better than the national benchmark in the literature of 70%." In some cases, you may want to report on significant improvements even if you have not yet reached your eventual goal—for example, "Report turnaround time reduced by 50% to 30 hours, nearing our goal of 24 hours." Please try to report at least one improvement in process and one improvement in outcome.

Your quality meetings in the next month would be a good opportunity to reach consensus in your area about the *two or three key accomplishments* that you would like recognized in the annual quality report.

Please return your list by no later than [date].

Thank you for your help. All departments will receive a copy of the final report, outlining a broad range of improvements. In case of questions, call _____.

In addition, a simple query should be made to every department and team leader at the end of each year, requesting highlights of the past year's significant achievements (Figure 12.5).

One of the most satisfying responsibilities of a PI director—though certainly not the easiest—is that of producing the annual PI appraisal or self-assessment. In this document, you will have the ability to celebrate and compliment the organization and its staff for all their dedication and accomplishments of the year. You will have the pleasure of pulling together all of the good

FIGURE 12.6

Annual performance improvement program assessment

Each year, you must evaluate the PI program's overall progress and determine if there is room to make improvements. The following checklist is designed to help ensure that your PI program has performed well. The goal is to be able to answer each question in the affirmative and to produce documents, data, reports, storyboards, and committee minutes demonstrating compliance.

Yes	No	
❑	❑	Are the hospital's PI priorities defined clearly?
❑	❑	Is there a stated methodology for choosing PI projects and goals?
❑	❑	Are clinical leaders in all disciplines involved in the PI program?
❑	❑	Do you compare the hospital's current performance to its past performance, to other organizations' performance, to best practices, and to national literature or guidelines?
❑	❑	Have you incorporated basic quality monitoring and quality control throughout the hospital, as appropriate?
❑	❑	Can you demonstrate that the hospital monitors and evaluates all of the JCAHO's functions and dimensions of performance as appropriate?
❑	❑	Do you use consistent planning and reporting formats and structures as much as possible?
❑	❑	Do you use an external reference database(s) to compare data?
❑	❑	Have you documented the governing body's discussions of quality indicators, performance measures, results of comparisons, and rationale for pursuing or declining to pursue improvement opportunities?
❑	❑	Do all PI teams and department leaders receive appropriate facilitation, coaching, leadership, training, education, and technical and data management support?
❑	❑	Do all PI teams and department leaders produce summary reports, storyboards, or posters that concisely show how they used the organization's methodology effectively to improve performance of a process that was important to customers?
❑	❑	Do all PI teams and department leaders produce quality data and information?

news, all of the impressive improvements, and all of the self-congratulation that everyone needs so much—and that you are often too busy to recognize regularly throughout the year.

The annual appraisal should answer three primary questions:
- How did we actually improve the processes and outcomes of patient care and support services this year?
- To what extent did we meet the goals we set for ourselves?
- Did the program itself fulfill all pertinent regulatory and accreditation standards (e.g., routine reporting, all functions addressed, and leadership responsibilities fulfilled)?

Figure 12.6 provides a checklist that will help you assess the quality of your PI program. Figure 12.7 contains an outline of a typical PI program annual assessment.

Chapter 12

FIGURE 12.7

Outline of a performance improvement program annual assessment

To comply fully with the PI standards, it is essential that you compile an overview of the improvements implemented during the year (see Figure 12.3). In addition, this assessment should discuss how well the program is managed (see Figure 12.4). In other words, your annual assessment should document how you assessed the structure and process of the PI program and the outcomes the program was able to produce.

Remember, your annual assessment should be approved at all levels of the hospital, up to and including the board of directors. It should be carefully reviewed to ensure that all JCAHO-mandated functions and measurements are discussed; if this is ensured, the assessment will be extremely helpful during the triennial survey to demonstrate and lead surveyors directly to compliance data.

See the following outline of a typical annual PI assessment.

Outline

  I. Definition of quality and performance in our hospital and this year's PI goals

 II. Highlights of hospital-wide major PI accomplishments

III. Highlights of major external recognition of our PI program, such as regulatory and accreditation commendations, media attention, awards

IV. Departmental accomplishments

   This should include a modest number of significant quality and performance improvements and/or accomplishments. Remember to focus on quantitative and objective measures where possible. In addition, whenever possible, data should be accompanied by interdisciplinary statements.

 V. Overview of the hospital's chosen PI model

Once the annual appraisal is completed, it should be provided to the governing body for review and approval. This is an opportunity for a celebration of the hospital's successes and to identify improvement opportunities and goals for the coming year. The annual appraisal thus serves the JCAHO compliance requirements, but it also stimulates further enhancement of the PI program by recognizing and rewarding staff who have been responsible for its success. It may even be incorporated into your hospital's incentive compensation program.

The annual appraisal is also a wonderful introduction to your program for new management and professional staff. It gives them a sense of your pride in your program and shows them the kinds of improvement you seek to implement.

External rewards for an outstanding performance improvement program

Since the creation of the national Baldrige award in the late 1980s, there has been a notable increase in the number of forms of external recognition available to U.S. businesses for development of impressive quality and business excellence.

The Baldrige award criteria are not replacements for the JCAHO standards, but they can be of value in conducting a truly rigorous evaluation of the hospital's focus on its leadership, human resources, process improvement, customers, and outcomes. (There are several books available that map the Baldrige and JCAHO criteria to each other.) The award has been opened to hospital applicants, with guidelines modified appropriately, and many state-level Baldrige look-alike awards have been created that also accept hospitals as applicants.

A few of the many awards currently involving some evaluation of quality include:

- National Committee for Quality Health Care Award.
- Voluntary Hospitals of America Leadership Awards.
- Marriott Service Excellence Awards.
- *USA Today*'s "Golden Cup" Award.
- The JCAHO Codman Awards, designed to recognize the use of process and outcome measures to improve performance. The awards are named after Ernest Amory Codman, MD, a physician who first defined clinical quality outcomes measurement in the early years of the twentieth century.

Notes

Appendix 1

Pre-Survey Checklist: Accreditation Requirements for Performance Improvement

Standard	Assessment Point	Yes	No	Example of Compliance	Notes
PI.1	Do you have an organization-wide approach that is consistently used for • Designing new processes? • Revising existing processes? • Measuring performance? • Making decisions about performance? • Improving performance?	❏ ❏ ❏ ❏ ❏	❏ ❏ ❏ ❏ ❏	Your PI plan explicitly applies to all patient care and support services, and all new and redesigned/improved patient care and support processes. The plan outlines an approach and process for planning and implementing quality measurement and improvement. You have evidence that PI is well understood in your organization; for instance, all staff use common terminology and are aware of what is being done to improve quality in their area of the organization.	
PI.1.1	Are PI activities in your hospital performed collaboratively?	❏	❏	Interdisciplinary teams work together on performance improvement projects, and on developing clinical paths and designing new processes; selected performance measures assess the quality of interdepartmental processes. Leaders, medical staff, and employees all use the same approach. Evidence of these activities can be found within specific departments as well as within cross-functional teams.	

Appendix 1

Standard	Assessment Point	Yes	No	Example of Compliance	Notes
PI.2 PI.2.1 PI.2.2	As you revise or design new processes, do you ensure that they • Are consistent with the hospital's mission and strategic goals? • Meet the needs of the customer(s)? • Are consistent with current clinical or business practices? • Include baseline performance expectations? • Consider inherent risks and any published data on the potential for sentinel events?	❏ ❏ ❏ ❏ ❏	❏ ❏ ❏ ❏ ❏	The hospital uses flow charts, focus groups, or comparative or benchmark data from other providers when developing new processes; pilot testing is used to introduce new processes; pertinent, focused measures test the efficacy of the new process over time.	
PI.3 PI.3.1 PI.3.1.1– PI.3.1.3	Do you systematically collect data • To gauge your current performance? • To measure improvement and document sustained improvement? • To identify opportunities for improvement? • On issues identified for more in-depth assessment? • To measure processes with inherent risk?	❏ ❏ ❏ ❏ ❏	❏ ❏ ❏ ❏ ❏	A review of the measures in place for this year provides evidence that you measure important processes to provide assurance that performance is acceptable, that interventions designed to improve processes are consistently documented with measures, that issues that should generate more intensive assessment are measured, and that an occurrence screening program monitors the incidence of processes with risk.	
PI.3.1	Does data collected to gauge performance consider the following: • The selection, patient preparation and education, performance, and post-procedure care for operative and other invasive or noninvasive procedures? • The ordering, administration, and impact of medication use? • The ordering, handling, and administration of blood, and the monitoring of blood use? • The use of restraint and seclusion? • Appropriateness of admission, discharges, and transfers? • Patient satisfaction? • Employee and physician views on performance and performance improvement activities? • Behavior management techniques? • Risk management activities?	❏ ❏ ❏ ❏ ❏ ❏ ❏ ❏ ❏	❏ ❏ ❏ ❏ ❏ ❏ ❏ ❏ ❏	A review of the current organizational measures shows that consideration is given to the scope and complexity of the services you provide, and measures have been selected to reflect this range of services. You can credibly explain how you have selected the mix and number of measures and show that new measures are added as changes are made to the scope of services. Financial, market share, and other measures that may be required by regulatory or accrediting agencies are considered in addition to clinical measures.	

Standard	Assessment Point	Yes	No	Example of Compliance	Notes
	• Quality control activities? • Infection control activities? • Success of approaches to pain management? • Other data important to the organization's performance?	❏ ❏ ❏ ❏	❏ ❏ ❏ ❏		
PI.3.1	Do you collect data on processes that place the patient at risk, including at least the following: • Medication errors? • Adverse drug reactions? • Operative and invasive procedures (e.g., surgery, cardiac cath., endoscopy, etc.)? • Administration of blood and blood products? • Use of restraint? • Use of seclusion? • Other services to high-risk populations (e.g., chemotherapy and radiation therapy)?	 ❏ ❏ ❏ ❏ ❏ ❏ ❏	 ❏ ❏ ❏ ❏ ❏ ❏ ❏	The hospital periodically collects and analyzes data on high-risk processes; results are presented to the hospital's quality improvement committee, and recommendations for improvement—if any—are acted on. The hospital compares itself to benchmarks and incorporates published findings when appropriate. Pay close attention to those indicators that are required. For those that the JCAHO has recommended that you consider, make sure that your documentation can support that you have considered these—for instance, your quality committee minutes include a discussion at the annual planning meeting.	
PI.4 PI.4.1	Do you systematically aggregate data and assess collected data using run charts, control charts, and other statistical analyses to determine whether a process is stable?	❏	❏	A control chart monitors time to the examination room in the emergency room and demonstrates that for 4 consecutive days, the time exceeded the upper control limit; assessment of the data showed that out-of-control days were the result of special cause. The relevant committee considered the data and made a determination of how to continue measuring and reporting.	
PI.4.2	Do you compare your hospital's performance data against • Its own past performance? • Recent, relevant references in the current literature?	 ❏ ❏	 ❏ ❏	Minutes from a planning meeting note that the decision to expand the emergency room was based on data that showed increased	

Appendix 1

Standard	Assessment Point	Yes	No	Example of Compliance	Notes
	• Benchmarks of best practice from other providers? • Interactive reference databases?	❏ ❏	❏ ❏	waiting times by shift and by day of week compared with the previous year, an increase in patient complaints about delays during the same time period, and a comparison to national data in similarly sized hospitals. All hospitals currently have ORYX data and this is another item that should be regularly and thoughtfully assessed.	
PI.4.3	Do you conduct intensive assessments • When occurrence reporting identifies a potential or actual sentinel event? • When comparative data indicates a significant variance over time, from other providers or from the literature? • For unacceptable events, such as significant adverse anesthesia incidents, confirmed hemolytic transfusion reactions, preoperative/postoperative discrepancies, or significant adverse drug reactions?	❏ ❏ ❏	❏ ❏ ❏	A multidisciplinary team assembles to investigate a potential sentinel event and uses analysis tools, such as Pareto charts, fishbone diagrams, flow charts, control charts, or others, to determine the root cause(s) of the process failure. After analyzing the data, the team generates recommendations for changes to the process.	
PI.4.4	Do you have a procedure for performing a root-cause analysis that • Focuses on identifying system or process problems? • Documents recommendations and solutions for problems? • Includes a follow-up mechanism to evaluate the effectiveness of your actions?	❏ ❏ ❏	❏ ❏ ❏	A hospital uses the JCAHO format for performing a root-cause analysis. It uses the JCAHO grid (included in a booklet that the JCAHO provides free of charge to all accredited organizations, and also available on their Web site) to record the process. *Note: A hospital may use its own PI model, provided that the hospital analyzes all possible causes, including special and common causes.*	
PI.5	Can you demonstrate systematic performance improvements in your organization over the past 12 months?	❏	❏	PI projects demonstrate that your PI process is effective and measures demonstrate sustained improvement; leaders can describe how significant PI activities fit with the hospital's mission and strategic goals; reports to the governing body summarize significant improvements made within the organization.	

Reprinted from *The JCAHO Mock Survey Made Simple, 2000 Edition,* authors Kathryn A. Chamberlain and Candace J. Hamner. Copyright 2000, Opus Communications, a division of HCPro, P.O. Box 1168, Marblehead, MA. Revised by the authors of this book.

Appendix 2

Pre-Survey Checklist: ORYX Compliance

The Joint Commission on Accreditation of Healthcare Organizations details its ORYX/core measures program requirements in the Accreditation Participation Requirements chapter of the *Comprehensive Accreditation Manual for Hospitals*. Review these questions and examples of compliance, and prepare your own answers for surveyors. For more information, see Chapter 3.

ORYX Questions	Yes	No	Examples of Compliance with ORYX
1. Have you picked an approved system and at least six relevant clinical indicators?	❑	❑	You have selected the Maryland Hospital Association's Quality Indicator Project as your measurement system and have decided to collect data for submission to the JCAHO on six indicators. You have a signed contract and have tested the system for submitting data and receiving reports and can show that it is accurate.
2. Do you have the appropriate hardware and software, if necessary, to meet the requirements of your measurement system?	❑	❑	The measurement system requires that you have at least a 486 computer and a modem, and have installed the system's software items.
3. By first quarter 2000, did you begin to collect data on your most recent two indicators?	❑	❑	You have reviewed and understand the data requirements for your new indicators. You have begun to collect the data in the format specified by the MHAQIP.
4. Do you have documentation that ensures that the measurement system will submit your data to the JCAHO in a timely fashion?	❑	❑	Your contract with the measurement system states that the measurement system will submit the data on the selected indicators by the deadline specified by the JCAHO. You submit the data as required by the JCAHO. Each quarter, you receive reports from the system that mirror the information that the vendor has sent to JCAHO. You carefully check the accuracy of the report and share it with all relevant quality committees so that they can do an assessment of your performance compared to the vendor's benchmarks.

Reprinted from *The JCAHO Mock Survey Made Simple, 2000 Edition,* authors Kathryn A. Chamberlain and Candace J. Hamner. Copyright 2000, Opus Communications, a division of HCPro, P.O. Box 1168, Marblehead, MA. Revised by the authors of this book.

Appendix 3

Pre-Survey Checklist: Sentinel Events

Beginning April 1, 1998, the JCAHO has asked organizations to self-report certain sentinel events. If you choose to comply with this requirement and minimize the risk of receiving an accreditation watch designation, consider establishing a policy that addresses sentinel events. Review these questions and compliance examples to help you create your policy. For more information, see Chapter 10.

Sentinel Events Questions	Yes	No	Sentinel Events Examples
1. Do you have a definition of sentinel event that includes: • An unexpected event resulting in death or serious injury? • An unexpected event that carried the risk of death or serious injury?	❏ ❏	❏ ❏	As part of your policy on sentinel events, include a definition such as: This hospital defines a sentinel event as an unusual, unexpected patient occurrence that results in death or serious injury to the patient; or, in special situations, an event in which the break in process was so egregious that serious injury could have resulted to the patient, posing a threat to other patients if the problem with the process is not corrected.
2. Do you have a procedure for doing a root-cause analysis that: • Focuses on identifying system or process problems? • Drives the organization to discover the underlying cause(s) of the event? • Documents recommendations and solutions to solve problems? • Includes a follow-up mechanism to evaluate the effectiveness of your actions?	❏ ❏ ❏ ❏	❏ ❏ ❏ ❏	Use your own PI model, provided you do a thorough analysis of all of the possible causes, including special and common causes, or use the JCAHO format for performing a root-cause analysis. Note: If you choose to use your own PI model, you should put the results in the JCAHO format (see the JCAHO's free booklet about conducting a root-cause analysis that was sent to all organizations and the information at the JCAHO's Web site).
3. Do you have a JCAHO reporting policy regarding sentinel events that requires employees to report: • An unexpected event resulting in death or serious injury? • Abduction of an infant? • Discharge of an infant to an incorrect family? • Rape (by an employee or another patient)?	❏ ❏ ❏ ❏	❏ ❏ ❏ ❏	As part of your hospital policy on sentinel events, include the time frames for reporting, the criteria for inclusion in reporting, the time frames for conducting and reporting a root-cause analysis, and who is responsible to report. For example: The hospital will report within 5 days of the occurrence, or notification of the occurrence, any event that meets the JCAHO reporting criteria (list criteria). A root-cause analysis will be submitted within 45 days of notifying the JCAHO of the event. The director of quality

Sentinel Events Questions	Yes	No	Sentinel Events Examples
• A hemolytic transfusion reaction? • Surgery on the wrong body part or the wrong patient? *Note: The JCAHO states that a hospital should voluntarily report these events, but does not require reporting. Please check JCAHO literature for full details. You should also consult with your own legal staff and senior management on the pros and cons of reporting.*	❏ ❏	❏ ❏	improvement/risk management will be responsible for determining which events the hospital will report.

Reprinted from *The JCAHO Mock Survey Made Simple, 2000 Edition,* authors Kathryn A. Chamberlain and Candace J. Hamner. Copyright 2000, Opus Communications, a division of HCPro, P.O. Box 1168, Marblehead, MA. Revised by the authors of this book.

Notes

Bibliography

Books

Berwick, Donald. *Curing Health Care*. (San Francisco: Jossey-Bass, Inc., 1990).

Brassard, Michael. *The Memory Jogger Plus*. (Madison, WI: Joiner Associates, 1989).

Carey and Lloyd. *Measuring Quality Improvement in Healthcare: A Guide to Statistical Process Control Applications*. (New York: Quality Resources, 1995).

Carr, Maureen P. and Francis W. Jackson *The Crosswalk: Joint Commission Standards and Baldrige Criteria*. (Oakbrook, IL: Joint Commission on Accreditation of Healthcare Organizations, 1997).

Cesarone, Diane. *Assess for Success: Achieving Excellence with Joint Commission Standards and Baldrige Criteria*. (Oakbrook, IL: Joint Commission on Accreditation of Healthcare Organizations, 1997).

Crosby, Philip. *Quality Is Free: The Art of Making Quality Certain*. (New York: Penguin Books, 1979).

Goal/QPC and Joiner Associates, Inc. *The Memory Jogger: A Pocket Guide of Tools for Continuous Improvement and Effective Planning*. (Methuen, MA, 1994).

Goal/QPC and Joiner Associates, Inc. *The Team Memory Jogger*. (Methuen, MA, 1995).

Hartzler, Meg and Jan E. Henry, *Team Fitness: A How-To Manual for Building a Winning Work Team*. (Milwaukee, WI: ASQC Press, 1994).

Joint Commission on Accreditation of Healthcare Organizations. *A Pocket Guide to Quality Improvement Tools*. (Oakbrook, IL: Joint Commission on Accreditation of Healthcare Organizations, 1992).

Joint Commission on Accreditation of Healthcare Organizations. *Comprehensive Accreditation Manual for Hospitals*. (Oakbrook, IL: Joint Commission on Accreditation of Healthcare Organizations, 1997).

Joint Commission on Accreditation of Healthcare Organizations. *Exploring Quality Improvement Principles: A Hospital Leader's Guide*. (Oakbrook, IL: Joint Commission on Accreditation of Healthcare Organizations, 1992).

Joint Commission on Accreditation of Healthcare Organizations. *Framework for Improving Performance: From Principles to Practice*. (Oakbrook, IL: Joint Commission on Accreditation of Healthcare Organizations, 1994).

Bibliography

Joint Commission on Accreditation of Healthcare Organizations. *Implementing Quality Improvement: A Hospital Leader's Guide.* (Oakbrook, IL: Joint Commission on Accreditation of Healthcare Organizations, 1993).

Joint Commission on Accreditation of Healthcare Organizations. *Process Improvement Models: Case Studies in Health Care.* (Oakbrook, IL: Joint Commission on Accreditation of Healthcare Organizations, 1993).

Joint Commission on Accreditation of Healthcare Organizations. *Transitions: From QA to CQI-Using CQI Approaches to Monitor, Evaluate, and Improve Quality.* (Oakbrook, IL: Joint Commission on Accreditation of Healthcare Organizations, 1991).

Joint Commission on Accreditation of Healthcare Organizations. *Using Quality Improvement Tools in a Health Care Setting.* (Oakbrook, IL: Joint Commission on Accreditation of Healthcare Organizations, 1992).

Kohn, Linda T., Janet M. Corrigan, and Molla Donaldson, eds, Committee on Quality of Health Care in America, Institute of Medicine. *To Err is Human: Building a Safer Health System.* (Washington, DC: National Academy Press, 2000).

Leebov, Wendy and Clara Jean Ersoz. *The Health Care Manager's Guide to Continuous Quality Improvement.* (Chicago: American Hospital Publishing, 1991).

Leebov, Wendy. *The Quality Quest: A Briefing for Health Care Professionals.* (Chicago: American Hospital Publishing, 1991).

Melum, Mara Minerva and Marie Kucheris Sinioris. *Total Quality Management: The Health Care Pioneers.* (Chicago: American Hospital Publishing, 1992).

Opus Communications. *The JCAHO Survey Coordinator's Handbook.* (Marblehead, MA: Opus Communications, 1997).

Rosander, A. C. *Deming's 14 Points Applied to Services.* (Milwaukee, WI: ASQC Press, 1991).

Scholtes, et al. *The Team Handbook.* (Madison, WI: Joiner Associates, 1988).

Spath, Patrice, ed. *Innovations in Health Care Quality Measurement.* (Chicago: American Hospital Publishing, 1989).

Journals

Journal for Healthcare Quality, National Association for Healthcare Quality, Glenview, IL.

Perspectives, The Official Joint Commission Newsletter, Joint Commission on Accreditation of Healthcare Organizations, Oakbrook Terrace, IL.

The Joint Commission Journal on Quality Improvement, Joint Commission on Accreditation of Healthcare Organizations, Oakbrook Terrace, IL.

Quality Management in Health Care, Aspen Publishers, Frederick, MD.

Annotated List of Healthcare Quality-Related Web Sites

http://acsi.asq.org
American Customer Satisfaction Index

http://www.ahcpr.gov
The Agency for Health Care Policy Research

http://www.apqc.org
American Productivity & Quality Center
"The American Productivity & Quality Center is in the business of improving your organization through education, training, benchmarking services, action research, networking opportunities, publications, and other media. A wide variety of information is available from the Center on these topics: benchmarking, knowledge management, measurement, customer satisfaction, and productivity and quality."

http://www.healthcare.org/
American Society for Quality—Health Care Division
"Members are providers of healthcare and services, supporters of those providers, and interested others."

http://www.hcia.com
"HCIA is a leading healthcare information content company that develops and markets clinical and financial decision support systems used by hospitals, integrated delivery systems, managed care organizations, employers, and pharmaceutical manufacturers. The company's databases and products are used to benchmark clinical performance and outcomes, profile best practices, and manage the cost and delivery of healthcare."

http://www.dhhs.gov
Federal Department of Health and Human Services

http://www.ismp.org

The Institute for Safe Medication Practices (ISMP) is a nonprofit organization that works closely with healthcare practitioners and institutions, regulatory agencies, professional organizations and the pharmaceutical industry to provide education about adverse drug events and their prevention. The Institute provides an independent review of medication errors that have been voluntarily submitted by practitioners to a national Medication Errors Reporting Program (MERP) operated by the United States Pharmacopeia (USP) in the USA. The Institute is a U.S. Food and Drug Administration (FDA) MEDWATCH partner and regularly communicates with the FDA to help to prevent medication errors. The Institute encourages the appropriate reporting of medication errors to the MEDWATCH Program.

ISMP is dedicated to the safe use of medications through improvements in drug distribution, naming, packaging, labeling, and delivery system design. The organization has established a national advisory board of practitioners to assist in problem solving.

http://www.jcaho.org

"The Joint Commission evaluates and accredits more than 15,000 healthcare organizations in the United States, including hospitals, healthcare networks and healthcare organizations that provide home care, long-term care, behavioral healthcare, laboratory, and ambulatory care services. An independent, not-for-profit organization, the Joint Commission is the nation's oldest and largest standards-setting and accrediting body in healthcare."

http://www.quality.nist.gov

Malcolm Baldrige National Quality Award

http://www.cdc.gov/nchs/default.htm

National Center for Health Statistics

"The mission of the National Center for Health Statistics (NCHS) is to provide statistical information that will guide actions and policies to improve the health of the American people. As the nation's principal health statistics agency, NCHS leads the way with accurate, relevant, and timely data."

http://www.ncqa.org

"The National Committee for Quality Assurance (NCQA) is an independent, not-for-profit organization dedicated to assessing and reporting on the quality of managed care plans, including health maintenance organizations (HMOs)."

http://www.nih.gov

Federal National Institutes of Health

http://www.nnlm.nlm.nih.gov/nnlmlist.html

National Network of Libraries of Medicine

"The purpose of the National Network of Libraries of Medicine TM (NN/LM TM) is to provide health science practitioners, investigators, educators, and administrators in the United States with timely, convenient access to biomedical and healthcare information resources."

http://www.cost-quality.com

The Quarterly Journal of Cost and Quality

"The journal's focus and mission is to provide healthcare leaders with a reference that blends clinical and financial information in a practical and readable format."

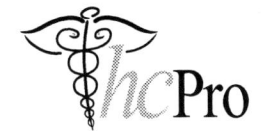

Related Products from HCPro

Books

The Compliance Guide to the Medical Staff Standards—Winning Strategies for Your JCAHO Survey, Second Edition

By Richard E. Thompson, MD

Explains and examines the JCAHO medical staff standards and offers advice on how to

- avoid common mistakes that can adversely affect JCAHO accreditation
- prepare your medical staff for survey using 18 easy-to-implement tasks
- educate medical staff leaders, the hospital's survey coordinator, and physician leaders on the JCAHO's medical staff standards

Conscious Sedation, Anesthesia, and The JCAHO

By Dean F. Smith, MD

Polls show that most JCAHO surveyors ask hospitals about their conscious sedation policies and procedures. Are you prepared to answer confidently?

Dean F. Smith, MD, an anesthesiologist and authority on the JCAHO's requirements for conscious sedation and anesthesia, has authored the definitive guidebook on one of the most confusing accreditation issues for hospitals.

Conscious Sedation, Anesthesia, and The JCAHO is the only book of its kind. It explains, once and for all, when the anesthesia standards apply to sedation, and it provides:

- practical tips on development of conscious sedation policies
- field-tested sample policies that you can use as models
- useful advice on assessing your organization's compliance with the JCAHO's anesthesia standards
- tips on survey preparation
- guidance on how to credential and privilege practitioners involved in anesthesia and conscious sedation

> Related Products

Don't risk a Type I Recommendation. *Conscious Sedation, Anesthesia, and The JCAHO* will tell you when the anesthesia standards apply and what you need to do to comply. When it comes to conscious sedation, this book is the only tool you'll need.

Continuous Quality Improvement for Health Information Management
By Jennifer I. Cofer, RRA, and Hugh P. Greeley
Continuous Quality Improvement for Health Information Management is written for health information management (HIM) professionals who want to take a proactive approach to improving and maintaining quality, and who will not settle for less than peak performance.

Formerly known as *Quality Improvement Techniques for Medical Records,* this new edition addresses the latest strategies for making continuous quality improvement (CQI) part of your department's culture. And it introduces more CQI tools and techniques than ever before.

This practical resource includes an introduction by James H. Braden, the innovative system director of HIM at the Detroit Medical Center, and it offers

- all new case studies that bring CQI theory to life and address some of HIM's most challenging issues
- more CQI tools—and step-by-step descriptions of how to use them
- a complete, easy-to-use CQI implementation plan
- a comprehensive CQI inservice kit for staff education
- an updated resource guide
- tips to help readers and their staffs put CQI to work in their HIM departments

First Do No Harm: A Practical Guide to Medication Safety and JCAHO Compliance
Contains up-to-date information on the current state of medication use in hospitals and what, specifically, the JCAHO requires. You'll get practical advice on meeting the TX.3 standards and sample solutions for common problem areas.

Information Management: The Compliance Guide to the JCAHO Standards, Third Edition
Offers you a straightforward analysis of JCAHO's IM standards and includes detailed, practical advice on how to develop an information management plan, improve your medical records, and prepare your facility for JCAHO survey interviews.

j-mail: JCAHO Survey Prep E-mails for the Whole Staff
By Candace Hamner, RN, MA
Preparing staff for survey the old fashioned way can be a daunting task, especially in larger hospitals or multi-hospital systems. How do you reach everyone involved in your survey in a timely, cost-efficient manner and still educate staff with one-on-one detail? It's easy when you use *j-mail*.

j-mail lets survey coordinators use e-mail to prepare staff for survey. The disk contains 12 months' worth of field-tested survey prep quizzes, hints, tips, and strategies. Send the e-mails out as is or customize them to your own organization. The accompanying guidebook also offers practical tips and strategies to help survey coordinators launch e-mail training campaigns. It's never been easier to educate and prepare more people at one time for a JCAHO survey!

The JCAHO Mock Survey Made Simple, 2000 Edition
By Kathryn Chamberlain, CPHQ, and Candace Hamner, RN, MA

Written by two JCAHO survey coordinators, this convenient workbook provides 27 comprehensive checklists for pinpointing problem survey areas before they turn into Type I recommendations. The pages are perforated, user-friendly, and ready to hand out to your survey teams to make your mock survey a snap to coordinate.

The JCAHO Survey Coordinator's Handbook, Second Edition

Designed to walk you through the complicated survey preparation process from start to finish, it offers easy-to-understand guidelines, tips, and other valuable suggestions designed to help you and your organization successfully meet JCAHO requirements. With this handbook's practical, step-by-step advice, you'll learn how to

- design and implement a survey preparation plan tailored to your organization's needs—even if you're on a tight schedule
- assess your organization's compliance problems and develop realistic, easy-to-implement solutions
- successfully train your staff for all the JCAHO's required compliance areas
- select your survey preparation teams and orient them to their responsibilities
- review the quality of your medical records, policies and procedures, and other JCAHO-related documents
- prepare for survey using the included tasks, forms, and other helpful tips for success

The JCAHO Survey Coordinator's Handbook will help you successfully manage every facet of the preparation process.

The JCAHO Troubleshooter: Best Policies, Practices, and Model Documents for Survey Success
By Steven Bryant, John Rosing, MHA, FACHE, and Brenda G. Summers, MBA, MHA, MSN, RN, CNAA

Written by JCAHO survey consultant with years of experience, *The JCAHO Troubleshooter* offers a collection of the best policies and documents to achieve and demonstrate compliance with the most challenging JCAHO areas.

This comprehensive handbook covers the most common "trouble spots" in every chapter of the *Comprehensive Accreditation Manual for Hospitals (CAMH)*.

Some sample policies include:

- Advance directive policy
- Restraint and seclusion policy
- Sentinel event policy
- Medical records completion policy

You can also customize your own policies and documents with the user-friendly software!

Related Products

Leadership: The Compliance Guide to the JCAHO Standards
By Richard Schmidt Jr, LD, LLM, and Mary Becker, RRA, MBA
Provides you with detailed interpretations and advice on how to comply with each leadership standard and other related standards. You'll learn to address the other leadership groups—the board of directors, the medical staff, the administrative team, and hospital management—and direct them in their leadership roles as defined by the JCAHO's standards.

Patient and Family Education: The Compliance Guide to the JCAHO Standards, Second Edition
By Joan Iacono, RN, MSN, MBA, and Ann Campbell, RN, MSN
Examines all standards for hospitals related to current patient and family education and explains them in simple, practical terms. You'll learn how to develop a patient and family education program that meets the needs of your organization and its patients and, in addition, how to avoid Type I recommendations.

Ready, Set, JCAHO! Questions, Games, and Other Strategies to Prepare Your Staff for Survey
By Candace J. Hamner, RN, MA
Ready, Set, JCAHO! was created to make the job of survey preparation easier. This book provides universal techniques for helping everyone be better prepared and more at ease when survey day arrives.

This book presents simple, easy, and entertaining ways to disseminate essential information to staff throughout your organization. From quizzes and games to theme days and contests, *Ready, Set, JCAHO!* offers traditional and nontraditional training approaches. The book contains 100 questions that cover eight different focus areas:

- Human Resources
- Patient Care
- Leadership
- Patient Rights
- Management of Information
- Performance Improvement
- Patient and Family Education
- Safety

This versatile new book is a great tool:

- DEMYSTIFY the survey preparation process and take the fear factor out of the survey equation
- SIMPLIFY your training activities
- BUILD awareness and enthusiasm as your hospital readies for survey
- PREPARE your entire hospital staff for survey easily and economically

Restraint and Seclusion: Improving Practice and Conquering the JCAHO Standards, Second Edition
By Jack Zusman, MD
Dissects and analyzes the JCAHO's new standards relating to restraint and seclusion in clear, concise language. This book examines the pros and cons of restraint use, presents ideas for improving patient care in your organization, and discusses issues that relate specifically to seclusion.

Newsletters

Briefings on JCAHO
Everyday, thousands of readers rely on *Briefings on JCAHO* to bring them the information needed to succeed in the accreditation process. With Briefings on JCAHO we not only tell readers what the JCAHO standard changes are, we also explain how to comply with them. From reporting on the latest changes in the survey process to advising how to meet JCAHO standards and scoring guidelines, Briefings on JCAHO is key. We make sure to tell readers what the JCAHO doesn't!

With *Briefings on JCAHO*, readers receive the latest information on

- sentinel event policies, legal concerns, and how to conduct a root-cause analysis
- ORYX and what core measures will mean
- problematic restraint and seclusion standards
- preparation strategies for triennial and random unannounced surveys
- how to prevent the most common Type I findings
- and much more

Some free subscriber benefits include

> **E-mail Chat Group**—network with peers through "BOJ Talk" our e-mail discussion group where readers can network with their peers
> **Fax Express**—whenever news happens that just can't wait, subscribers receive the pertinent information by fax so they'll always be the first to know
> **Survey Monitor report**—every quarter, this report tells you what surveyors are emphasizing

Briefings on Hospital Safety
Advises hospital safety committees on how to meet the challenges of effective safety management. This newsletter provides safety committees with crucial information and offers guidance on how to improve safety in a hospital by preventing costly problems before they happen. All of the regulators are covered: JCAHO, OSHA, EPA, NFPA, FDA, and NRC.

Briefings on Patient Safety
Created exclusively to help health care professionals avoid adverse and sentinel events—and work through damaging circumstances should they occur—this newsletter shares best-practice informa-

tion regarding sentinel event prevention, performing root-cause analyses and developing organizational policies/infrastructures to support root-cause analysis and adverse event prevention.

Readers receive the latest on

- advice on root-cause analyses and quality improvement techniques
- case studies on adverse and sentinel events
- tips on how to comply with JCAHO, FDA, HCFA, and state regulators
- how to enhance patient safety
- implementing error reduction systems
- how to train medical staff and other department managers
- how to design safer patient-care systems

Some free subscriber benefits include

"BOJ Talk"—our Internet discussion group where readers can network with their peers
Fax Express—when late-breaking news happens that just can't wait, subscribers receive the pertinent information by fax or e-mail so they'll always be the first to know.
Special Reports—Whenever a new regulation is enacted that needs further explanation, our expert writers gather the necessary information and compile a Special Report.

For additional information or to order these and other products, visit us online at www.hcmarketplace.com or at www.complianceinfo.com. Please contact us at:

Opus Communications
PO Box 1168
Marblehead, MA 01945
Toll-free telephone: 800/650–6787
Toll-free fax: 800/639–8511
E-mail: customer_service@hcpro.com